Being Dad

Being Dad

For dads-to-be and the women who love them

SAM HOLT & TROY JONES

A&U

First published in 2010

Allen & Unwin
83 Alexander Street
Crows Nest NSW 2065
Australia
Phone: (61 2) 8425 0100
Fax: (61 2) 9906 2218
Email: info@allenandunwin.com
Web: www.allenandunwin.com

Cataloguing-in-Publication details are available
from the National Library of Australia
www.trove.nla.gov.au

ISBN 978 1 74237 126 9

Internal design by James Cooper, Double O Design
Index by Puddingburn
Set in 11.5/14.2 pt Adobe Garamond Pro by Bookhouse, Sydney

15 14 13 12

Printed and bound in Australia by Griffin Press

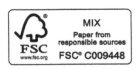

The paper in this book is FSC® certified.
FSC® promotes environmentally responsible,
socially beneficial and economically viable
management of the world's forests.

Contents

Prologue
The *Being Dad* story

You're probably wondering who the bloody hell are these blokes who have penned this book and why don't they have a string of impressive qualifications after their names? Well, for starters, we don't have any qualifications that are impressive, at least none our publisher thought worthy! We aren't medical, health care or relationship experts. Let's be honest, on paper we are pretty unimpressive. Why then have we written a book on pregnancy, birth and parenting?

Having been through the experience of having our first kids we sat around wondering why we had been so poorly advised about what was in store for us as dads. In the information age, how is it that so much vital information about becoming parents had bypassed our collective inboxes? As we explored our experiences and failings together it became apparent that the pregnancy and parenting world just wasn't catering very well to the needs of men or couples. Given the staggering amount of media on the subject for women, why was it that the male and relationship perspective was missing?

After reviewing parenting books, films, websites and other information we decided to do some market research by putting eight new dads in a room, plying them with copious amounts of beer and forcing them to talk about pregnancy and birth. After three hours of emotionally charged conversation we realised that blokes typically don't talk to each other about their experiences—but when they do it's incredibly beneficial. Our test dads laughed, cried and sat in quiet rapture as they listened to one another talk for the first time about becoming a father and the change in the dynamic of their relationships. What was even more amazing was that women loved watching blokes talking about pregnancy, birth, fatherhood and relationships. Like the early settlers striking gold, we had our Eureka moment. By getting blokes to open up about all these topics we could actually help both men and women make a happier transition from couple to parents.

Being Dad, a series of films by dads, for dads (and also for women to peek behind the thick velvet curtain that hides the male mind), was conceived. Armed with a shoestring budget, we set off around the country and interviewed groups of new dads and a few 'real' experts about pregnancy and birth. Eerily, nine months later our new baby was born: *Being Dad* the DVD. What we've learnt through making the initial film in Australia and subsequent films in the US and the UK is that by uncovering the world of pregnancy from a male's perspective we have inadvertently helped women and couples make pregnancy and birth more enjoyable and happy.

This book is a distillation of the information, experiences and advice we have gleaned from the real parenting experts around the world: everyday blokes who are fresh from their first go around in the pregnancy and birth caper. We aren't about pushing an agenda and we don't represent any organisation or viewpoint. Our only aims are to help men become great dads, to help women understand their partners better, and to help couples make a happier transition into parenthood. We've taken our knowledge of the male mind and applied it to making pregnancy and birth a happier experience, a less bumpy ride, for a couple.

We haven't tried to create an ultimate guide to pregnancy and birth, and we apologise in advance for not covering issues like multiple births, special needs children, same-sex parenting and single parents.

Making *Being Dad* taught us a great deal about men, women and couples. By watching the *Being Dad* films or reading this book you can learn, as we all do, from people who have been there and done it. It's about people sharing the quintessential human experiences: life, birth and love. We hope this book helps couples think outside the box, be aware of their choices, be more understanding of each other and become happy parents. Because if we've learnt one thing, it's that happy parents make happy kids.

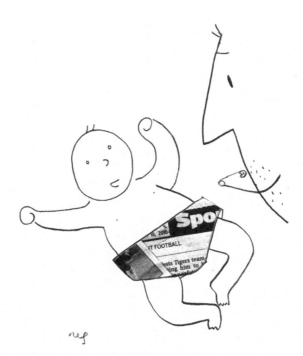

Introduction

FOR H⚥R

'Not another bloody book on pregnancy!' we hear you say. Well, sort of . . . it is another bloody book on pregnancy, but in this one we are also going to look at how each phase of pregnancy and parenting affects your bloke and your relationship with him.

How will pregnancy, birth and parenthood affect him and how will it affect your relationship? What issues will he be dealing with, what will be going through his mind and how can you help him be more supportive during pregnancy and become a better dad faster? In today's politically correct world we're not sure what we're supposed to call your man, the one who will one day be called 'Daddy'—so let's just call him your partner.

The pregnancy part of this book is primarily for you. It's designed to help you get your man into baby mode by understanding what makes him tick and what can be done to get him prepared, motivated and excited about fatherhood. Every chapter has a section for you and a section for him. You might like to read his chapters too just so you know what we are telling him. As the book moves into birth and beyond it becomes a little more focused on him but, again, if you read his chapters you'll get a good understanding of what we are doing to help you.

We've loaded this book with all sorts of secrets, tips and lists to help him, you and your baby. But all that is not a substitute for a parenting class or a normal pregnancy book (for you); this book is a companion, to help you make sense of the bloke you care about the most.

For the *Being Dad* films, we interviewed hundreds of dads from around the world as well as experts and celebrities to uncover one of the great mysteries of the world: the male mind. Generally we found that the great secret of what is going through the male mind can be answered with one word: nothing. Seriously. On a conscious level, not much goes on in there from one minute to the next. In such a complicated, fast-paced, info-rich world, please understand how much skill it takes to keep the male mind empty. Great effort and enormous leaps of faith and logic are required to do it, and we pride ourselves on it. It's not easy. But remember, to say it is empty is not to say that it is not complicated. The average man has all sorts of well-honed tricks to keep that cognitive space straightforward and able to concentrate on the footy. Once you recognise it, you can see it everywhere. It usually manifests itself in the form of 'I'll think about it when . . .' or 'I'll think about it if . . .'. We like to call it denial, and Australian men, even when compared with men in the US or the UK, are the undisputed kings.

Pregnancy and birth are among the most complicated, surreal, long-term and life-changing concepts for men to understand. After surveying and interviewing hundreds of intelligent, successful Australian men, the number one emotion that is felt immediately upon the birth of their first child is surprise. Despite nine months of pregnancy, pregnancy tests, morning sickness, hormones, baby showers, baby kicking, ultrasounds, birth classes, books and everything that goes with it, he is still surprised that a baby has been born. Such is the ability of the Aussie male mind to keep nebulous concepts at bay. He's tried very hard to concentrate on the status quo, because the life he's about to walk into is a total mystery to him. You, along with this book, can help him start to shine a light into the darkness of that future mystery.

All of this might suggest that we don't want to know what's happening. That we're reluctant about having a baby. That we are the stereotypical male sitting out in the waiting room or the pub across the road while you get on with the challenges of birth. Not true. We desperately want to be involved, to be good dads and to help you. It's just that no one tells us what we are in for, we don't read, and very few self-respecting Aussie males talk about pregnancy with their mates until after the birth, and even then it's with those who have already been through it.

And to be fair, who knows what could happen if we actually let ourselves stop and think about something?

Along with the guys from *Being Dad*, we are here to help you help him by understanding how to work with the void, how to penetrate it, when to reap the benefits of keeping it empty and when to get through to the real thoughts, fears and hopes that are actively, but subconsciously, being held at bay.

Think of this book as your roadmap to your partner's mind. It will enable you to get from conception to parenthood and beyond with your relationship and sanity in one piece. Even better, we think a better understanding of each other through pregnancy and birth will bring you much closer as a couple. There's not much that is more honest, real and binding than having a baby, and we think it's something that can be enjoyed, rather than feared.

We're here to help. And as an added bonus, it stops us thinking about the things that we should be thinking about . . . so it's a win-win.

FOR H⚉M

The secret to surviving pregnancy, birth and beyond, our friend, is to try to understand the mind of the pregnant woman. You may think, 'Forget it, *ce n'est pas possible!*' You may say you'll never understand women, especially pregnant ones. But if you can't, how can you make the treacherous journey ahead with our sanity and marriage intact? That's where we come in.

Your pregnant partner is an even greater mystery than the woman you knew before. She's about to be internally assaulted by a heady cocktail of hormones so intense you'll wonder if she's truly possessed. Wonder no more: she is—or at least, she will be.

Let's get another thing straight from the get go: there's no point denying it, you're either about to start trying for kids or you've already kicked a procreation goal and you're going to become a dad. Think about it, and believe it: in the not too distant future a little person will emerge from your partner. Either way things are going to change in your life, but not for the worse.

As Aussie males we are born with the denial gene. If there was a world championship in denial we would win the trophy every four years without breaking a sweat. This book has been expertly crafted to help you stop putting things in the 'denial pile' so that you can genuinely enjoy pregnancy, birth and the first year of being a dad. Millions of blokes have gone before you, made the mistakes and learnt the hard way. This book is the distillation of their successes and failures.

We promise to keep things on a need-to-know basis, provide valuable advice to make your life easier and arm you with enough knowledge to keep you in the good books and one step ahead of trouble. Just by reading this book you're doing more than most of those who have come before.

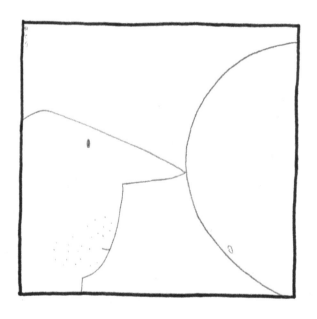

We know that the idea of reading a book on pregnancy and birth is as daunting as a paper cut to the eyeball, so bear with us. We've done our very best to keep it informative yet entertaining. Without further ado, it's on with the show.

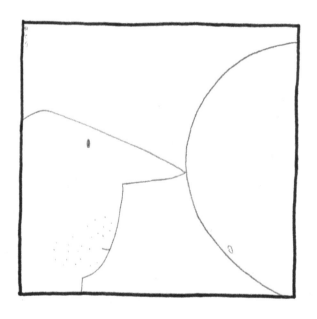

Chapter 1

Conception or misconception?

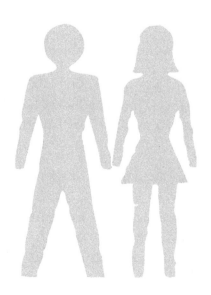

FOR H*R

Perhaps conception should really be called misconception, as there are many misconceptions about conception. For some, getting pregnant is as easy as tying their shoelaces, but for others it's a much more challenging and emotionally draining experience. The one thing we have noticed, however, is that like most things in life, getting pregnant is easier when you're not trying.

Many of our parents omitted the 'big talk', though some mates, oddly, refer to what must have been a very explicit and highly rating *21 Jump Street* episode, which seems to have triggered mums across the country to explain the birds and bees to their slightly too old sons. At the time, it all sounded pretty straightforward, but, as we can no doubt agree, unfortunate disasters throughout the many subsequent years attest to the fact that life is far more complicated than anything in a 1980s teen romp.

Wildlife expert David Attenborough probably knows how birds and bees feel about conception but we doubt they have the same issues we do:

- Do birds and bees get drunk, have unprotected sex and get pregnant accidentally? If so, do they care?
- How many female birds who are on the pill (or some other form of birth control) get pregnant every year?
- How many bee couples argue about when is the right time to have baby bees?
- How many male birds start worrying about having to pay for school fees before conception?
- Do female birds know when they are ovulating or sneakily buy ovulation kits from Woolies?

- Does a female bird who is trying to get pregnant become upset when her bird friends and EVERYONE else around her falls pregnant but she doesn't?
- Are there IVF clinics that birds and bees can attend?
- Do male bees get an SMS or bee-mail telling them to be back at the hive early because Mrs Bee is ovulating?

We've taken the most natural of interactions between a man and a woman and turned it into a systemised, scientific process. No wonder the world is a mess . . . we've forgotten that making babies is supposed to be fun, enjoyable and natural.

Other than navigating a wedding, conception is often the first major hurdle faced by couples. How can you get across this minefield successfully? It is important to understand how your partner will view conception, how important communication is during the process and what you can do to overcome typical man-problems that may arise.

Trying to get pregnant—the first 12 months

You've heard the saying 'It takes two to tango'? Well, we've tried to tango and it definitely takes two . . . plus some skill, patience and teamwork if you want to do it well. Baby making is no different.

Getting pregnant is emotional for men and women for completely different reasons. The aim should be to keep it as simple as possible, at least for the first 12 months. How can you keep him on the job at the crucial times without turning what should be everyone's favourite pastime into an experience to rival milking time at the dairy?

Having reviewed hundreds of hours of interviews with new dads, we've come up with a very typical range of issues that arise during conception that highlight the differences between men and women when it comes to baby making.

Month 1—Let's have a baby, baby

> Whenever we talk about having kids he says he's as ready as he'll ever be. I want him to be certain and to want them as much as me.

SHE SAYS

> She is always asking me how much do I really want kids. I do want them. I'm not sure if I'll ever feel like I'm 100 per cent ready. I do feel I'm as ready as I'm ever going to be, but that doesn't seem good enough. I'm not really ever 100 per cent sure about anything... let alone becoming a dad!

HE SAYS

Translation

There are exceptions to every rule, but it's probably safe to assume he'll never feel 100 per cent ready or have no reservations. You might have to settle for him being 'as ready as he'll ever be'. Many women say that at some point in their life having a child becomes all consuming. We've never heard a man say that—have you? If he's not 'as ready as he thinks he will ever be' you could be in for a long road ahead so it is important to discuss the realities of fatherhood.

Month 2—Let the baby making begin

> He tells me he wants kids but whenever we've had sex he seems reserved, or not into it. I think he's scared of being a dad and I'm not sure he's ready.

SHE SAYS

> *It's really strange, but when she is ovulating and I know that we are having sex to get pregnant I start getting freaked out. I've spent my entire life trying not to get women pregnant and it just feels unnatural to be trying to get her pregnant. I'm not sure if it's the pressure or a bit of fear. I do want to have kids but this baby making is weird—it's like teaching a cat to bark. I've tried explaining it to her but she just doesn't get it.*

HE SAYS

Translation

He may find baby making strange for the first few months. Trying to get you pregnant is a significant change of approach and it may feel unnatural or even wrong for some. Keeping it simple and not applying pressure is important.

Month 3—My temperature and mucus consistency is right ... game on!

> *Whenever I mention that I'm ovulating he goes all strange and our sex life is getting strained. I know exactly when I'm ovulating because I'm using ovulation kits and a thermometer, and I test the consistency of my mucus. He should be happy that we are doing it at the correct time ... right?*

SHE SAYS

> *Every month our bathroom becomes a laboratory. Ovulation kits, thermometers and God knows what else. I'm starting to dread the ovulation window. Why do I even have to know when she's ovulating? Can't she just want to have sex as often as possible throughout the month? It's pretty tough getting turned on when she starts talking about mucus consistency and internal temperature—are we supposed to be having sex or doing a chemistry assignment? I'm feeling pressured and I'm having problems feeling turned on.*

HE SAYS

Translation

We understand the benefits of ovulation kits and we're sure they can be very useful but your man does NOT need to know when you're ovulating. When you make the combined decision to get pregnant you need to start ramping up your sex life. Try to have sex consistently, not just when you're ovulating. By all means use the kits, but please hide the kits and thermometers and just get it on! It may help you to know when you'll be ovulating so that you can make sure you have sex on O-day, but the rest of the month should also involve lots of loving. Don't make him feel like an inseminator. Keep him in the dark about when you're ovulating and he won't feel so pressured.

Month 4—Period = tears

> I've been trying for four months to get pregnant and every time I get my period I get really upset and frustrated. He is very unsupportive and just keeps telling me not to worry. I don't think he really wants me to get pregnant, but he should know how important it is to me.

SHE SAYS

> Bloody hell, I dread the pregnancy testing each month. I pray she's pregnant so we don't have to go through the days of tears and emotional turmoil. I just don't get the rush—she knows that it can take up to a year or more. It's going to happen, so I just wish she'd relax. I hope she gets pregnant SOON—I can't take the drama!

HE SAYS

Translation

Be realistic—give yourselves a minimum of 12 months. The minute you start freaking out about not being pregnant after a month or crying because one of the Spears girls is pregnant again he'll start getting scared. If you're freaking out, try not doing it around your man. He's not likely to get upset or to understand why you are, especially in the first year of trying, but that doesn't mean he isn't hoping like hell that you will fall pregnant quickly. Most importantly, try to be patient and remember that he does want you to be pregnant.

Month 5—Frustration central

> *I swear to God if Mike comes outside of me again when I'm ovulating I'm going to murder him.*

SHE SAYS

> *Sometimes I just get caught up in the moment and I'm enjoying having sex and not thinking about baby making. God help me if I forget to come inside her—I swear she'll castrate me if it happens again. She makes me feel so bad when it happens. Whatever happened to enjoying sex together?*

HE SAYS

Translation

When he wants to have sex or make love he doesn't want to be thinking about getting you pregnant. It's very important to enjoy your love-making—having sex just to get pregnant will alienate him very quickly. Mistakes happen and you just need to remind him that when you do have sex he needs to hit his marks. Mix it up when you're not ovulating, too. If he doesn't know when you're ovulating and when you're not, and it doesn't matter what he does with the batter, try talking up some more exotic moves—put the excitement and unpredictability back in the sex life for you both.

Month 6—The pain and strain of making babies

> *I texted him, asking him to come home early because I'm ovulating and he went to the pub on the way. I'm furious with him.*

SHE SAYS

> *Sex has become pretty methodical. I really feel she only wants me to have sex with her so she can get pregnant. I even got a text message the other day saying 'I'm ovulating don't be late home from work'. I've been finding excuses to not have sex just because it's becoming no fun at all... I guess I should talk to her about it.*

HE SAYS

Translation

When sex just becomes nothing but a baby making exercise it can be downright terrible for both of you. There is nothing worse than awful sex; it's worse than no sex at all! If you find yourselves in a sexual rut it's time to spice up your sex life to make you both feel sexy. Try buying some new lingerie and mixing up your normal operating style between the sheets. Use this time to re-invent yourselves and to explore some new options . . . you might be surprised at how much fun you start having. If he knocks you back, play with yourself in bed—no one likes to miss a party and it's sure to drive him crazy.

Month 7—The book says . . .

> *When I'm ovulating I want him to have sex three times a day. I also think we need to stop drinking alcohol, eat macrobiotic vegan food, sleep upside down and wear no underpants—at least that's what the books say.*

SHE SAYS

> *Who'd have ever thought that I'd not want to have sex three or more times a day? I'm feeling a bit overwhelmed by the pressure now and having sex three or four times a day is bloody hard. I think I'm shooting blanks!*

HE SAYS

Translation

You might need to be clever in how you schedule your sessions. Set your alarm for the middle of the night or early in the morning and he'll be so sleepy he won't even count that as one of the two or three you're looking for. Don't restrict yourselves to the bedroom and don't set alarms or schedule sessions in his Outlook calendar.

Month 8—To be able to come or not to be able to come, that is the question

> *Sometimes he says he just can't come. He's never had that problem before. I don't get it. What does it mean??*

SHE SAYS

> *I've never felt pressure to orgasm before. It normally happens pretty easily—unless I'm drunk. The pressure is such that sometimes it stops me from coming altogether...it's horrible and stressful. I'm fairly certain that if I applied pressure on her to come every time it wouldn't happen but that doesn't seem to matter.*

HE SAYS

Translation

He may not come every time you want him to, especially if your love-making has become systematic or stressful. Keep it simple, mix it up and take your time. Enjoy the ability to have sex when and where you want—once you do have kids all that will change for a while!

The most important points from all of this are:

- Keep having sex regularly during the month, not just when ovulating.
- NEVER mention the words 'ovulation kit', 'vaginal mucus', 'basal temperature' or 'ovulation'.
- Spice things up, explore some new frontiers—and most importantly, enjoy sex while you can!
- Be realistic. Getting pregnant takes time and he may not share your urgency.

So there you have it. On the surface he seems like an uninterested selfish prick, but he's just a typical bloke who hasn't yet realised the significance of the changes afoot. It's only early days in the parenting experience and already there seem to be many areas of possible conflict. Parenthood is an assault on your relationship, and the sooner you prepare for battle the better the war you can wage!

After 12 months, or when fertility problems arise

If you've been trying for 12 months or more it may be time to see your doctor and get fertility testing. By now you're both probably feeling emotionally drained. It's now time to pack your man off to the nearest clinic for a sperm test. We've looked at many studies, and it seems that males are responsible for couple infertility between 25 and 50 per cent of the time. That's a big window and it means that it's really worthwhile being tested, especially as around 70 per cent of male infertility problems can be treated.

Fertility issues bring with them a whole new range of emotional turmoil for him and for you. Your doctor is best placed to explain possible problems with the female and male plumbing—they can be many and varied. There is a great factsheet that can be downloaded from Andrology Australia at www.andrologyaustralia. org/library/MaleInfertility_FactSheet.pdf.

How will getting a sperm test affect him?

It may be that your man is embarrassed, worried or just nervous about having his sperm tested. The actual test itself is a doddle: one simply masturbates into a sterile cup. It can be done at home or at a hospital with an andrology lab and, yes, it is true—they do provide free pornography.

SAM: Along with millions of men worldwide I have done the test several times, and for me doing the test in a hospital was definitely one of the most surreal experiences of all time. I showed up for my appointment, was led to a room (that locks from the inside, which is a very good idea, as they say that the organ that works the hardest while masturbating is your ears). I was then shown where the 'reading material' was and told to try not to spill any, or use lubricants or saliva while milking the snake of its venom. As a fan of late 1970s styles, the reading materials were excellent. No articles.

Matching the 1970s feel was the unavoidable idea that I was replacing Chevy Chase starring in an unreleased sequel to *Fletch*. Once the feeling of awkwardness had passed, I quickly contemplated my situation. This was a fully sanctioned wank. Not just by my wife, but surreptitiously by my family, my friends, even the federal and state governments of Australia. This was to be no ordinary wank. If there was a baby rattling around somewhere in my plums, by gum, I would flush the little fella out. I was not doing this act of self-gratification for myself. This was for the country. This was for the Wallabies. I could practically hear John Eales urging me on.

Locking the door, with *Waltzing Matilda* ringing loudly in my ears, I leafed nonchalantly through some softcore 1970s (or very cheap 1990s) porn, and put in a seriously entertaining performance. I was tender. I was loving. I was finished.

Handing the specimen jar back to the lab technician, the attendant treated it like a wine connoisseur would a glass of Penfolds Grange Hermitage. Honestly, she held it up to the light, gave the jar a swill and made a little comment under her breath. I'm sure it was complimentary . . .

So the initial test simply isn't that bad, but some men do report that it can feel a little degrading. It's all in the mind. I say go for it. The tough bit is next.

The results

It was a very serious dent to my sense of masculinity when I was told that I had problems with my sperm. Many infertility issues can be treated, but there isn't much that can be done for those of us with low sperm counts, poor motility (how well they can swim) or poor morphology (the shape of the sperm). Every man and his dog told me that it wasn't my fault, that it happens to everyone and that it would work out in the end. Not one of them stopped me from feeling like a failure, though. Yes, there are sperm washes, artificial insemination and IVF, all of which can help you get pregnant, but that doesn't cancel the idea that your sperm are hopeless duds, a dying race or just too plain ugly to get a run with Charles Darwin's theories. The medical processes certainly don't stop you feeling that you and your boys are just not quite up to scratch.

*   *   *

If your man receives news that his little fellas aren't such great swimmers he may experience these feelings:

- Loss of masculinity.
- Loss at the prospect of not being able to become a father.

- Guilt—he may feel that you think of him as less of a man and that you can't have children because of him.

- Depression—if he doesn't feel he can talk to anyone about it.

We are all different and we all have different coping mechanisms, but what is important is that you recognise that infertility issues will affect him, as they would you.

That's your work done for the night. We haven't even got pregnant yet and you can already see the potential pitfalls ahead. He's not likely to think or react the way you would or as the way you'd like him to, but that's not necessarily a problem. Understand him and learn how to work with what you've got.

You can pass the book to him now or, if you really want to eavesdrop, keep reading . . .

FOR H♦M

So you thought baby making was going to be fun. The reality is that the time ahead may be—no, will be—difficult and stressful. You may get her up the duff on your first angry shot down range or you could be in for a long and emotional journey. You need to be prepared for any possibility. If you're serious about getting her pregnant you should eat healthily, exercise, give up smoking and not drink too heavily. You will probably already be very familiar with these steps, and may not like the sound of it all, but making an effort will help your chances and it will make you look serious in her eyes. If you need help, sing out . . . we know a place with excellent 1970s porn.

Fire in the hole and bun in the oven

For some people conception happens quickly; they are what we call (among other things) lucky bastards. For these blokes it is usual to feel surprised, scared and a bit cheated. Surprised that it happened so quickly, scared because you didn't think you'd have to really think about being a dad just yet, and cheated because you were hoping for a few months of unlimited sex. All you lucky bastards have our permission to skip to the next chapter. We won't tell anyone. You can pretend you're a really fast reader, not to mention fast breeder. Seriously, fast forward. We want to talk behind your backs. For everyone else, read on.

On the practice range for several months

For a fit and healthy couple the average time to get pregnant is around ten cycles (months, that is). Every month you have a 20–30 per cent chance of falling pregnant if all goes well.

For most of us mere mortals it will take some time and you may find yourself having to deal with a raft of emotions. After a few months of baby making attempts sex can become routine, systemised and stressful, so it pays to sit down before you start and plan how you're going to tackle this issue. Do you want to know when she's ovulating? Do you find listening to tales of mucus levels, internal temperature readings and ovulation windows titillating? Yes? OK, no more book for you. No? We're with you. Read on.

*   *   *

Many guys have told us stories about their wives becoming baby crazy once they start trying. Below is a list of common situations and some suggestions as to how best to deal with them.

She wants a statutory declaration that you're 100 per cent ready for kids

Many of us can never truly say we are 100 per cent ready. Personally, we're never 100 per cent sure about anything, including what beer we feel like at the pub. By being prepared to talk about issues such as finances (wills, health insurance, budgets etc.), maternity/paternity leave, life with a child, or anything like that, you will demonstrate that you're serious about kids. It's very likely you'll only be able to admit to being 'as ready as you'll ever be'—there's no need to feel bad about that.

It's all about being honest and clear with your communication: you love your partner, you want to have a baby, and you want to learn as much as you can about becoming a great dad.

When hugging is a man's best friend

There is some debate as to whether it's beneficial for a woman to stay lying down for a few minutes after you've ejaculated. It's certainly not going to hurt and it's a good opportunity to remind her that you're excited about becoming a dad or to talk her through your latest round of golf. She may want to hang upside down from the ceiling for an hour; if so, go grab a beer or nod off to sleep. You're not a bat, and your job is done. Well done, stallion.

She becomes obsessed with identifying when she's ovulating

It's one thing to be obsessed, it's entirely another to share that. Ask yourself (and her) why she is telling you. Will it affect your game in any positive way? Talk of ovulation kits, using thermometers to gauge internal temperature and an obsession with mucus consistency can arise. None of these makes us feel particularly aroused and we're sure we're not alone. We're not sure that men need to know exactly when their partners are ovulating; it seems to just increase the pressure. Commit to increasing your sexual activity to at least every other day and try to keep talk of ovulation windows to a minimum. Explain to her that you're happy to have sex as much as possible until she falls pregnant but that you want it to be about being together, not just about getting pregnant.

She wants a lot of sex in the ovulation window

It can be tough having to back up multiple times during the ovulation window. You'll be expected to orgasm every time and it's not always easy. Try mixing it up: different positions, rooms, times of the day, themes, wigs, role-plays—whatever it takes. Get creative and enjoy the fact that you're able to have loads of sex, because once the baby comes along things will change for a while. Work out what's best for you—every day or every other day. Just be sure to be open and communicate with your partner about how you're feeling. If you're having regular sex you're less likely to know which days are ovulation days and therefore feel less pressured.

The thought of trying to get someone pregnant is difficult

You've spent your whole life trying not to get women pregnant. Don't be surprised if at first it feels weird shooting live ammunition. Once again, if you don't know which days you're in the ovulation window you can keep throwing stones and not think about the consequences of breaking the glass.

We don't know quantum physics well, but we know period = tears

After a few months of trying she may start getting emotional when she gets her period. A typical bloke's reaction is to say something like 'She'll be right' or 'Don't worry, love, it will happen', but our research shows that what she really wants is simply for you to be sad too. If you're not, don't be frightened to pretend. Do not tell her to stop stressing and it will happen.

One of our favourite pieces of advice is that women are not designed to be understood, they are designed to be loved. Work with what you know about women, and don't try to convince them of what you think is logical or accurate. Empathise, play the game and live happier as a result.

Abstinence reduces sperm count

Studies show that abstaining from sex for seven days or more can reduce your fertility. This is yet another reason to keep on the job throughout the month, not just in the fertile times.

Sperm testing

If you've been on the job for six months or more, you'll win a few brownie points if you offer to have a sperm test. It's basically a fully federally sanctioned wank. All you need to do is go into your local hospital, view some free pornography and do what you do best. It's a touch embarrassing having to hand over the specimen jar, but let's be honest: it's nothing compared with what your partner will experience in pregnancy and birth.

Nine myths about baby making (for both of you)

1. Too much bike riding is bad for your sperm. Lance Armstrong has sired two kids even with testicular cancer. It's unlikely any man will do more miles in his entire life than Lance Armstrong in his pre-breakfast training session. Personally, we think Lycra should only be worn by professional athletes and therefore think bike riding is bad for the health of the rest of us.

2. The position you have sex in determines babies' gender. You're a 50/50 chance in any position, so go with what feels best. Our favourite Aussie joke on the topic: man and wife with their obstetrician. The man asks, 'What position will my wife give birth in?' Obstetrician, with a smirk on his face says, 'Most likely the same position that she conceived in.' Man remarks, 'Oh, with one leg out the window in the back of a taxi?'

3. It doesn't matter if the female orgasms. True, but if you believe that it's hard to see how you've stayed married this long.

4. Tight trousers cause infertility. So ask yourself, 'Why am I wearing tight trousers?'

5. Taking the pill means you can't get pregnant. Ninety-nine per cent of the time that is correct.

6. Masturbation reduces the chances of getting your partner pregnant. True, if you're masturbating in private, unless your sperm have feet.

7. Hanging upside down after sex increases the chance of sperm reaching the egg. Maybe, if you're a vampire.

8. The word 'mucus' is sexy.

9. You can't get pregnant outside the ovulation window. This is actually true but it can still be fun trying. We also would prefer to not know what an ovulation window is.

In summary, it's up to you to communicate, mix it up in the bedroom, be aware of her emotions and make the most of baby making so that it doesn't become a chore. How bad can it be? A free sex pass!! Remember, she wants you to be excited, committed and supportive. Now is a good time to get into the habit of all of these— when she does fall pregnant you're going to have to really step up!

Until now you've probably never imagined that some sex can be bad sex, but women have been aware of this since they first started out. Baby making sex can be truly awful for both of you if it becomes systematic and pressured. Given that the average couple takes over ten months to fall pregnant, it's worth setting some ground rules from the get go. Make it fun and enjoy the fact this may be the last time for a long time that it's just the two of you.

The online female language of being pregnant

For a giggle and a wide-eyed look at what is going on behind our collective backs, visit a few of the more popular mums' websites such as huggies.com.au or kidspot.com.au and have a read of the 'trying to conceive' community posts. This is where women like your partner are online talking about the trials and tribulations of trying to conceive and generally whingeing about you. It will give you a terrific insight into how seriously the girls take this baby making business. You'll also learn a new language. Much like hieroglyphics, it's practically indecipherable. Here are some of the modern phrases we have learned in our cyber travels. In truth, these are a bit like our teenage sexual adventures . . . a stab in the dark. We're not entirely sure, but think we're fairly close. Here goes:

LOL Laugh out loud

LMAO Laugh my arse off.

DH 'Dear husband' or 'dickhead'. We're not sure, but she's talking about one of us.

PG 'Pregnant' or 'Please God'.

BD Some reference to sex during ovulation window: 'bed down'? 'Be dicked'? Who knows? Maybe it's code for *Being Dad* (www.beingdad.com.au).

TTC 'Trying to conceive' or 'This time you c+nt'. (Probably the first.)

OPKs We're guessing it's 'ovulation (pregnancy) kits'. We hope so because we can't think of anything smart for the letters OPK.

BBT Basal body temperature. Nothing funny about that.

AF Aunt Flo/period/menses/menstruation/menstrual cycle.

BD Baby dance (a term for sex).

BFN Big fat negative. A 'not pregnant' on a digital test or no double line on a regular test.

BFP Big fat positive on a pregnancy test.

CD Cycle day. Cycle day 1 is the first day of your period. We always thought it stood for compact disc!

CM Cervical mucus. Why?? Please . . . no. Neither word is good. For crying out loud, don't put them together!

EWCM Egg-white cervical mucus. The obsession with mucus continues! Probably twice as bad as CM.

FMU First morning urine (the female equivalent of a PF, piss fat).

O'ING Ovulating.

POAS Pee on a stick. We assume pregnancy stick, not a stick in the garden where you enjoy peeing.

BFP We can't work this one out so we're going for 'bloody f+cking period', as in 'I'm not LOLing—I've got my BFP again and am not PG'.

CD 36 Calendar days 36 (since last period). Or maybe that's her rego number in case someone spots her about to drive off a large cliff.

OMG Oh my God!

TOO Took us a while to work this one out, but it is just the word 'too' in capitals.

As a great example of how this baby language operates, have a read of the paragraph below from a very popular website. We have NO idea what this woman is talking about, in fact we think she may be possessed. Note the reference to DH . . . OMG the poor bloke . . . LMAO.

> I have to say, ladies, that I agree with NOT trying so hard. No I'm not a mother, and it's only my third month TTC. The reason I feel this way is more because of the psychological ramifications that can take place when 'trying' so hard. The first month DH and I were trying, we were very lighthearted about it, no worries, not a huge deal. Yes I knew when I was ovulating but didn't really do anything else. Needless to say I didn't get PG BUT the way I handled it was a lot healthier than the way I handled it this month when I went full on charting, OPK, etc.

When I found out this month that I wasn't PG, I nearly came undone! Seriously! I cried b/c I totally convinced myself through 'phantom symptoms' that I was definitely pregnant. Not to mention that I almost threw a shoe at my DH when he was too tired to BD on one of the days during my fertile window! It just caused too much stress on the both of us and I felt like I was being TOO controlling over the situation. That being said, when you have sooo much control, and it doesn't work out the way you hoped, you fall harder than if you just left it up to God (as I believe) or to chance or whatever.

So for me, this will be the last month that I do the OPK, temping, etc. and then I'll take a break for a little bit. We won't stop BDing during peak times, but I won't micromanage. And if you think about it, you'll conceive when you're meant to conceive, so I'd rather be less stressed during the months or years leading up to it than completely going buck wild with CD counting DPO days, CM checks, early morning temps, etc. But again, that's just my opinion. If you can do this every day and not fall apart each month you get a BFN, then more power to you.

WOW . . . we didn't know 'micromanage' and 'pregnancy' could be used in the same sentence; nor did we think it would be possible to go 'buck wild with CD counting DPO days, CM checks, early morning temps, etc.'. Sometimes we're convinced the less we know the better, lads.

If there was a male equivalent entry on another website we think it would have read:

Me and the missus are trying to get pregnant. No joy so far but we'll just keep rooting . . . she'll be right. What about the cricket on the weekend!!

> ### Homework assignment for men
>
> Talk to your mates about their experiences with conception. You've probably never spoken to them about it before and you'll be surprised to learn that you're not alone in many of the emotions you're experiencing.

Are my boys swimmers? Fertility issues

If you've been trying for 12 months or more it may be time to see your doctor and get fertility testing. By now you're probably feeling emotionally drained and so is your partner. It's time to man up and head off to the clinic for a sperm test.

Fertility issues bring with them a whole new range of emotional turmoil for you both. Your doctor or web MD are best placed to explain possible problems with the female and male plumbing, but they can be many and varied. There is a great factsheet that can be downloaded from Andrology Australia at www.andrologyaustralia. org/library/MaleInfertility_FactSheet.pdf.

Chapter 2

Now that you're pregnant

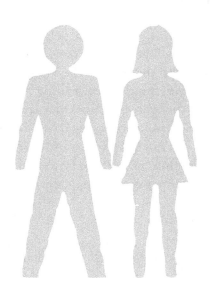

FOR H♦R

'OMFG I'm PG. Can't wait to tell DH!'

OMFG indeed. Does the F stand for what we think it does? Let's presume it does.

Either way, the bloke in your life is in for a severe shock. If you think about this for a moment, you'll see that you hold unimaginable power. The average man would savour this. He would enjoy the life-changing shock he holds in the palm of his hand, and would delight in planning the time and place to deliver it. The more surprised, freaked and shocked you are the better, he would think. He would know this is a marathon, and he would want to have some fun with the starting gun.

You probably won't go at it like this. You face a delicate, desperate feminine conundrum. How will he take this news? His immediate reaction will be a window on the soul. In the instant following the news, you will learn everything. There will be no time for reflection, composition or thought. Upon hearing one of the biggest, most surprising pieces of world-changing news his instant reaction will be ALL IMPORTANT. Did he want this? What are we going to do? Is he going to stay? Will he be a good dad? All will be revealed in his instantaneous reaction to this. What an enormous moment!!!

Right? Wrong.

So OMFG-ing wrong, in fact.

Understand this. Like the history of evolution itself, throughout the entire gambit of responses to this revelation, shock and surprise are the only genuine reactions. Not 'good shock', 'bad shock', 'joyous shock', 'hooray-my-life-will-be-heavenly shock' or 'I-didn't-want-this-and-my-life-is-ruined shock'. There is only one type of shock—best captured for all eternity and displayed on *Funniest Home Videos* for all to enjoy.

'Shock shock' is all you're going to get. Expect nothing more or less. Derive nothing from his reaction, NOTHING. He has no idea what you mean, what happens next, what that means, what to do, what you want.

Now, be fair.

Think about it: you had some idea you were pregnant, otherwise why did you buy the kit and wee on the stick? Not to mention you most likely had privacy and a few moments to compose yourself before moving on.

He, on the other hand, has the distinct displeasure of someone staring in his face (having just heard the bone-chilling phrase 'We need to talk'), looking for the slightest hint of any reaction to the biggest, most life-changing news he has ever heard. Don't read that as bad change . . . just change, which we don't react well to.

If this were a Ricki Lake show and we were African American chicks (ohhh, if only we were African American chicks . . .) We'd snap our fingers in a Z motion. We don't know why, but we think that applies here. Uttering something like the phrase 'girlfriend'.

Let's pause for an important Ricki recap.

In Chapter 1 we established that the male mind is a vacuum—a unique space in which it seems nothing exists, the laws of gravity are defied and weird happenings are afoot. We've come to appreciate that despite his shortcomings he really does have your best interests at heart and wants to have kids with you. However, we've also recognised that you're going to have to provide as much support to him as to the other baby in your life.

In this chapter we'll examine how to break the news to him and what thoughts will be whirring in that vacuum that sits atop his shoulders. It may come as a surprise that he will exhibit anxiety about becoming a dad. It shouldn't . . . why would it? Are you anxious? So is he, simple as that.

We will also look at the importance of re-evaluating your relationship with him, getting to know each other again and preparing your relationship for the changes ahead.

He's going to be a dad!

From the moment you discover that you're pregnant you are already a mum and he is already a dad (yes, that's a frightening thought). Sure, in his mind 'mini-him' is only the size of a Tic Tac and doesn't even have fingers or toes but you are both now responsible for providing a safe haven for the baby to develop and prosper in for the next nine months. Yes, that's right, you're BOTH responsible. He needs to look after you so you can look after the baby.

Girls (this part is written by Sam—he is alarmingly comfortable talking to women in the first person and adding emoticons to emails), we need to start getting him thinking like a dad. You both need to understand that from this point on you're a family, and the dynamic between you will change. By understanding what goes on in the male mind you can get him involved, make him feel he's part of the pregnancy and get him acting and feeling like a dad and family man.

Many dads talk of the shock to their system at the birth of their first child. The vast majority of us men sail through the pregnancy without really preparing ourselves for the changes that lie ahead. This need not be the case for your fella!

Passing on the big news

Telling your DH that you're officially pregnant can be one of the happiest days of your life, but terrifying at the same time.

OK, yes, we are blokes. And run of the mill blokes, too. But we think understanding it is a pretty simple exercise. Assume for a moment it's a similar emotion your man may have experienced when he asked for your hand in marriage. He'd been dating you for years, spoken many times about getting married, asked your father, knew the answer would most likely be yes, and was excited . . . but terrified to the point of irreversibly damaging his trousers. The fear of rejection can be enough to turn even the burliest of blokes into a sweating, bumbling mess.

You're probably the same: hoping that he's going to be jumping for joy at the news, but slightly terrified he's going to freak out and board the next plane to Guatemala.

As you're reading this book the chances are that you've planned this pregnancy and have been actively trying to conceive, so you think that he has at least some idea that it's possible you could be pregnant this month. Think again.

Our surveys show that even if you have been trying for a year or more to get pregnant, the primary emotion your man is likely to experience is still shock. Much like a bear going into hibernation, the typical male will go into denial until the baby literally emerges into his life. Not that this is a bad thing or an indication of anything, it is merely typical. Even the most loving, excited dads-to-be have no idea what the phrase 'Honey, I'm pregnant' actually means for them.

For this reason we recommend performing all pregnancy tests alone. The shock to his system may be such that he doesn't provide you with the instant source of affection and joy that you may be looking for. On the flip side if it's you who's in shock and needs some quiet time, sitting on the lavvy with your head in your hands, he's likely to be extremely confused. Test away in private or with a girlfriend if you need reliable support.

Don't think that priming him with subtle hints before you do the test will lessen the shock. You know the type of things we're referring to: 'I'm late', 'My breasts are sore', 'I'm so tired' and even 'I think I might be pregnant'. These phrases are only likely to cause a mild heart flutter (mainly because he heard the word 'breasts') as they rattle through his vacuous grey matter—he is putting great effort into not thinking about these things. And he's doing well. You have quite an adversary here.

Feel free to shock him—it's your privilege. Just don't expect too much in the way of a response. Read this first, OK?

> Remember! Pregnancy is a three-way street.

Pregnancy has long been the domain of women—and rightly so. Like any wedding day which revolves around the bride, pregnancy has always focused on women. We believe that's why men sail through the three trimesters in a world of denial: no one helps them, no one asks them, and it seems to them that no one much cares. The bloke in this situation is in real trouble . . . no one ever told him anything. Not his dad, not his mates. And you know he never read anything about it.

If we had $24.95 for every time we had a bloke come up to us and say, 'Mate, I saw your DVD . . . LOVED it, but when my missus thrust the video in my face, I would have done just about anything to avoid watching it,' we'd be rich. It's a desperate situation. When he says, 'I'll think about it when the baby gets here,' he actually means, 'I do not want to think about this until the baby comes out.' As we know that's way too late, but that is his plan. And even if people did tell him (which they actually most likely did), his brain took over and nothing actually was heard.

So when the big moment has arrived and it's time to pass on the news, think about doing it in a way that involves him from the start. Everything we've heard from women suggests that they don't want the pregnancy to be just about them. His excitement, connectedness and involvement enhances your experience, right?

If you can't hold it in and need to tell him straight away, here are a few ideas:

> 'Honey—you're going to be a dad!'
> 'Honey—we're pregnant!'

OK, so they both suck, but what do you want from us? You know him better than we do. And remember, no matter what happens, no matter how you phrase it, no matter what he is really thinking, his reaction will be shock and should never, ever, ever be judged as if it was from the rational heart.

If you can hold the news in and work in a bit of humour and fun, we have some ideas for you. Your first pregnancy should be a fabulous time, full of excitement—a time to enjoy each other's company before the baby comes along. It's important to remember that pregnancy isn't a disease and birth isn't (usually) a medical emergency. Why not introduce some fun from the very beginning? Here are a few ways to break the news to your man:

1. Create your own beer. There is a fabulous website called Brewtopia (www.brewtopia.com.au) where you can create custom beers. Simply pick out his favourite beer variety and then design your own label which announces the news. The beer can be delivered inside a week and you can fill the fridge with it for when he gets home one night.

2. If there is a DVD he's been dying to watch or one that is his favourite, suggest a quiet night in with your favourite takeaway food and a bottle of wine. Get him settled on the couch and discreetly slip *Being Dad* into the DVD player and see how long it takes him to realise what's happening. Make sure you pause it when he twigs and resume once he's come to.

3. If he's mad for a particular sport or team, buy a kiddie's jumper or piece of equipment (like a mini cricket bat or tennis racquet) and put it on the bed with a note saying that his baby can't wait to wear it/use it.

4. Treat it the way he treated the marriage proposal. Think of a way that really suits him and reinforces the good things about becoming a dad. This baby is a person he will love forever and will desperately want to be mates with, boy or girl. In the weeks after the birth he'll be thinking of 21st speeches in the shower . . . get him thinking like that.

5. Blurt it out and film it.

Engaging him from the first moment is like saying, 'Hey big fella—you're in this too.' Let him panic if he wants to. Let him ride the rollercoaster that is the experience of the first-time dad. If you can detach your own fears from the moment and be confident that your man will get there in the end, you can enjoy his flustery, blustery happy panic and look back on it and laugh in days to come.

Don't give him the opportunity to feel that you will be doing all the work for the next nine months. He needs to appreciate the important role that he will play in ensuring that you and the baby—and he!—are healthy and happy.

His reaction

The male mind has not much knowledge or experience to grab on to in the freak-out stages here. The bloke mind desperately searches for a problem to solve and a detail to concentrate on. Like those early DOS computers with the green screens and the flashing cursor, his brain will just sit there waiting for something to process:

```
C://DOS/Pregnant
C://DOS/
C://DOS/Blink
C://DOS/
C://DOS/WTF?
C://DOS/Pregnant
C://DOS/
C://DOS/Windows has encountered a problem and must
restart
```

During restart, where pretty much the only parts working are the eyelids, kidneys and heart, the main part of his brain will be processing data like:

'What did she say?'

'OK. What do we do now?'

'How could this happen?'

'Oh, yeah, that's right . . . he he . . .'

'I'm not old enough to be a dad!'

'I'm not rich or mature enough to be a dad!'

'I'll never play golf again. What's going to happen to my handicap?'

Research has shown that some men are able to process the news highly effectively and demonstrate genuine delight, joy and exuberance. If you have such a specimen, report him to the local university for further research. Our theory is that these men are either in touch with their humanity or—much more likely—very good on their feet.

Regardless of his reaction, if you've been talking about having kids (and he wasn't vehemently opposed) he will be delighted once the news has sunk in. It may be exciting or frightening for you both initially, so be prepared for his initial reaction to not live up to your expectations. Just don't expect much from him yet.

What are men really concerned about when it comes to parenting?

Men's concerns about parenting change during the pregnancy. At first they can't see real signs of the baby so it's more about intangibles like finance. As the baby starts to show and his brain fully comprehends what's occurring, the fears and concerns take on a more physical and emotional aspect.

Men go through a smorgasbord of worries as the trimester pass, from finances to upgrading the car, from facing up to the in-laws (yes, we had sex!) to the birth. We give you a complete analysis of your partner's state of mind trimester by trimester on page 47.

Trust us that there's a lot of worrying for nine months. Men are fixers by nature. If there's a problem we want to find a solution—as long as it's not in an instruction booklet (we don't want to find a solution that someone else has already discovered!).

Pregnancy delivers many issues and problems that can't be fixed. Pregnancy also can't be controlled. The loss of control plus the unpredictability can make men feel very uncomfortable, and can even lead to depression and serious anxiety. Our ability to bottle up our emotions means that we are not naturally good at coping with this huge change. This is where you and your ability to communicate come in.

You've broken the news—what's next?

The most important thing for you and your partner to do throughout pregnancy, birth and beyond is to reaffirm and continue to work on the love and respect you have for one another. Many first-time fathers feel detached, non-players in the process of pregnancy. It could well be how their dads felt—it's your job to make him feel part of the team.

'Why,' we hear you say, 'should I need to look after him as well as the baby?' The answer is simple: your brain is better wired to cope with relationship building and in the majority of cases women play the larger role in ensuring that relationships stay on track. Relationships are difficult at the best of times. Introduce a life-changing event such as pregnancy and birth, throw your routine into chaos and you have the makings of a relationship crisis. By crisis we don't mean impending disaster, we mean simply something major that warrants your attention.

There has been much research conducted into the elements of successful relationships through the parenting life stage and they all point to the same conclusion: working on your relationship, redefining your expectations of each other and spending time together before the baby comes are all vital for relationship success.

Here's a sobering fact: 10 per cent of couples break up during their first pregnancy and 30 per cent within the first two years of parenthood. Those statistics alone mean that you should together examine where your relationship is at and where you want it to be nine months from now.

Once the news is out and blood flow has resumed to his brain, take a few days to bask in the glory of your achievement. His boys can swim, you're growing a baby and you've both entered a new dawn of maturity. You're now on the same playing field as your parents—life is about to change. Then you can start talking to him about your relationship. You can plan for the future, and delve into each other's fears, anxiety, wants and needs.

Pregnancy is about growth and development, not just of your baby but of your relationship. Two becomes three and the road ahead becomes a relationship minefield. When you do that successfully, you'll find real happiness.

Think about it. Change management is something companies, sporting clubs and governments spend millions of dollars on every year. And they do this why? Because people hate change and companies know how disruptive it can be to business and earnings. Unfortunately, we give very little consideration to what effects pregnancy and birth will have on us as individuals and as a couple. There's an expectation that everyone will be cool with everything. There's no guidebook or expensive suit-wearing boffins there to help you through this. It's up to you guys—welcome to Parenting 101.

Sam Bittman and Sue Rosenberg Zalk, authors of *Expectant Fathers*, state: 'Pregnancy seems to ignite in all people their greatest fears and spark their most secret smouldering hopes.'

Planning for what's ahead

To give your relationship the best possible chance of survival it's a very good idea to get to know each other again. If you're like most couples you've probably been busy having a great time, working hard and enjoying the dwindling/never-ending days of your self-indulgent youth. Are you still the same people you were when you fell in love? Have your hopes and goals shifted over the years? How well do you really know each other? When was the last time you sat down and talked about your feelings for one another, your hopes and dreams for the years ahead—or whatever it is that floats your boat?

Wouldn't it be useful to know what your partner is thinking and to understand the male approach to pregnancy and relationships? He probably has deliberately not stopped to think about it! We think success relies on you understanding that he wants your relationship to be strong, wants to show you he loves you, but may not be much chop at effectively expressing that.

> The relationship you had with your partner before pregnancy will be different from the one you'll have during pregnancy. And your relationship during pregnancy will be different again from the one you'll have after your baby is born.

Get out the highlighter, or hand over the book to him now and we'll tell him what he can expect to feel in the coming months and how to handle those emotions. We'll also convince him of the need to re-evaluate your relationship and plan for what's ahead by better understanding one another. Once you've taken care of your relationship you'll have a great foundation for the perfect pregnancy, and for him being the perfect birth partner and dad. Just like the Year 9 boy reading the Dolly Doctor segment of the girl's teen magazine *Dolly*, feel free to read this but we advise caution. Chortling and disrespect may be unavoidable.

FOR H♦M

Holy shit, Batman—you're going to be a dad! Don't worry.

After days, weeks, months or even years of trying it has probably still come as a great surprise that you may actually be a dad in nine months. First, congratulations and second, it's OK, you'll be fine. Mates will be there, beer still tastes like beer and life rolls on. Boys' nights/weeks away are still on the cards—but you have to do some work to earn them AND you have added a string to your bow of life.

The way the news was broken to you will determine your reaction. Did she do the test in private or were you present? Either way there is a life-altering moment as you nervously await results of the disposable pregnancy test or as you try and compute the words 'Honey, I'm pregnant.' Time stands still, the world stops spinning and your life flashes before your eyes.

If we knew how to develop iPhone applications we'd create a pregnancy test app that allowed you to pee on your iPhone and record your reaction as it came up with the results. Granted, sometimes positive news can be far from good news for those people wanting to get pregnant, but it would still be a winner and the resulting videos would be guaranteed to collect the major prize on *Funniest Home Videos*.

Here's a quick low-down on common reactions:

1. SHOCK. Your system is going to hit the DENIAL button repeatedly, but repeat after us, 'I'm going to be a DAD.' Say it as many times as you can to yourself each day until it starts to sink in.

2. Your main question—'What happens now?'—is entirely normal. We both asked it and wondered it for years. Don't

worry. No one knows, including your missus. Honestly, you're in it together, and she is only a few steps in front of you. The answer is, relax. This is a VERY long, normal, healthy process. Stay informed, pay attention and understand that this is one of the biggest moments in her life to date (and she's not even in denial!). Make sure she enjoys it as much as possible. You have more control over that than you think. Remember your school formal? Don't be one of those shit blokes who sulks in the corner, slowly but surely ruining her night. Let's be honest: this is a major life achievement for your partner, and even if you're not feeling it yet put on a big smile and your dancing shoes, be a great guy and make sure she enjoys it.

3. You'll need money, maturity and masculinity. Yes, you can manage these three Ms and you'll be fine. There is something simple (but a little boring) you can do right now: contact a financial planner and get things like your insurance and wills in order. Your partner will feel better, and you'll be covering all of the bases. This is an important thing to do, so get on to it.

4. A wave of emotions, anxiety and fear—don't worry, it's completely normal to be thrilled one minute and crapping your pants the next. We'll get to the emotional mumbo jumbo later, but just remember it's OK to feel freaked out! It's OK to not be freaked out. It's OK to be not exactly in touch with reality. Just keep reading, breathing, smiling and nodding—and things will be OK.

Your missus is about to be swamped with a cocktail of hormones and bodily changes that will transform her from the woman you know to an at times cranky, tired, emotional and maternal being who will have you scratching your head or pulling out your hair one minute and feeling more in love with her than ever the next.

It's confusing, frustrating and downright impossible to know what's in store for you when you wake up tomorrow.

Even though it's kind of surreal, and on the face of it not much has changed, you have to start to focus on the concept that you're a family now. It's no longer you and the missus, it's the three, four, five or more of you—depending on how many nippers she has on board. (We hope that insurance you bought in point three covers heart attacks.) It's important to start realising that the woman you married is about to change, as are you and your relationship. Pregnancy is an opportunity to grow and develop individually and together—it can and should be a time of great happiness and excitement. You need to be prepared to work on your relationship, to strengthen the bonds that have kept you together so far so that you can make it through to the other side.

Connect with a mate who has just been through it and ask him the hard questions.

We are now going to look at common emotions felt by all guys when it comes to pregnancy. We'll talk about coping strategies for your emotions, and look at why it's important to start thinking like a dad and at what you can do to make your life easier, make your partner happy and provide the best possible environment for junior.

We've got it easy!

A quick look around the animal kingdom is enough to make you feel glad you're a Homo erectus. (For those of you still stuck mentally in Year 9, you'll notice two possible jokes there. Homo and Erectus. Ha ha, OK, we get it. Let's move on.)

Some other species have it pretty tough. Some male members of the insect world are devoured by their missus after they have inseminated them. Let's be honest, there probably have been some girls you'd gladly have slept with even if it meant being killed and eaten by them afterwards, but these days a cold beer or a nap is a much more enjoyable post-coital activity. That being said, at least male spiders don't have to change nappies.

Then there is the male seahorse, who is really in trouble: once his little lady seahorse has her eggs fertilised, she literally dumps them on his back and says, 'Look after these until they hatch, love, I'm off to party with the girls!'

On the face of it, we have the right end of the evolutionary pineapple. Once you've done the job it's nine months of having a designated driver and enjoying your dying days as a (somewhat) free and easy bloke! Or is it?

The reality, gents, is that you actually have a pretty important role to play for the next nine months. There is a saying among the midwifery community that 'A mum's job is to carry the baby, the dad's job is to carry the family.' By this they mean that it's up to us to be supportive, emotionally available and committed (or to literally carry your wife and baby around with you—I'd like to see the engineers at Baby Bjorn design that sling!).

This may not be as easy as it sounds, because most of us blokes want little more for their future with their kids than to be great mates with our children. We want an honest, open, loving friendship with well-adjusted kids. It's just that that journey starts sooner than we think. Too many blokes think (or hope) it really starts when the kid is old enough to start swimming lessons or kicking the footy in the backyard.

But first, and for one of the last times ever, let's get back to blokeland first and take a quick peek into the closet that we like to keep closed—the one with the word 'emotion' emblazoned across it. Sorry, but we have to. (If you bought this book and now you buy a copy for a mate you're allowed to skip this part.) We are regular Aussie blokes about to recklessly use words like 'emotion', 'feel', 'research' and 'duffle bag'. We sincerely apologise in advance.

What can you expect to feel?

There has been plenty of research done on prospective fathers and their emotional duffle bag. We've read plenty of it and it's quite enlightening and reassuring to know that what we went through—and what you're probably going through—is completely normal.

You probably know pregnancy goes for nine months. (Unless you're married to an elephant—it's 22 months! Tip: we also do not recommend mentioning anything like that fact to your wife. There is no possible way you can say 'elephant' and 'pregnant' and emerge with the point you were trying to make intact.)

Each three months is known as a trimester. Trimester 1, or T1 as women like to call it, is conception to three months and so on. We will expand on all of these in further chapters but here is an overview of emotions you're likely to encounter.

Trimester 1

- Money and finance, job security, mortgage payments—the big Kahuna himself.
- Your space—the first frontier.
- Your car's life expectancy post-birth.
- Your relationship—is it strong enough?

Trimester 2

- The in-laws—you're going to be seeing a lot more of them!
- Weight gain—yours and hers.
- Sex—will you ever get any again and will you want it?
- Responsibility—can you handle it, will you be a good dad?

Trimester 3

- Paternity—is it yours? Seriously!
- Health—hers and the baby's (miscarriage, birth defects etc.).
- Coping with the birth, cutting the cord, holding a baby, bringing the baby home, how to interact with a baby, how much does a baby sleep . . . so many questions, so little time remaining!
- Your ability to be a good dad/the type of dad you'd like to be.

As you can see, there will be plenty going on for you in the coming months. In the next few chapters we will look at the changes to your partner and the baby as the pregnancy progresses, but for the time being think about your relationship, how it will change and what you want from it in the future. Once you've addressed that you can start enjoying the next nine months.

She says/she means

Pregnancy is a relationship minefield. But we, your experienced brethren, can help you survive. Think of us as the evolution of man in an Xbox 360 kind of way. Many men have fallen so that you may have the following information. Think of us as the last saved point in *Call of Duty 4*. We know that there is a metaphorical baddie with a metaphorically massive bazooka around the next corner that could blow your metaforical, motherflippin' head off. You need to appreciate that the raging hormone levels in your partner will mean she's not always even vaguely logical. This section will help you translate some of the verbal rocket-propelled comments that may come your way.

She says	She means
I want to go and look at nursery items—you don't have to come.	*Come or else.*
I'm really tired. Can you cook dinner?	*She's exhausted; baked beans won't do.*
I have morning sickness	*She feels like she has a terrible hangover that does not go away by lunchtime.*
I'm going to the doctor today for my first check-up.	*We are going to the doctor today.*
I wonder if the car will be big enough?	*I just drove part a 4WD dealership and want one.*
We need to start thinking about wills etc.	*Find out about will, you lazy shit.*
Is my bum looking bigger?	*I feel fat already; give me a compliment, please.*

(Proceed with extreme caution. This is a challenge. Make sure you save all your points so far before attempting this one.)

Remember, the game you're playing during pregnancy is a totally new game. The game rules you're familiar with will change quickly and unexpectedly. Your partner's files have been corrupted by a serious virus: hormones. Game play can become highly unpredictable and volatile.

You're a dad now. It's time to put down the Xbox and pick up a will kit, a Babies Galore catalogue or just give your little lady some extra loving. In the next few chapters we will explore trimesters 1, 2 and 3 and prepare you for the birth. For now, put the book down, go for a run and clear your head. There are great times ahead, you're not alone and everything will be OK—trust us!

Chapter 3

Trimester 1

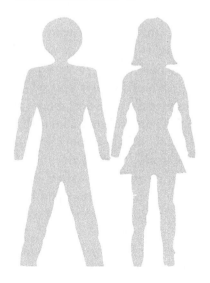

FOR HER

If you're like most first-time pregnant mums you've probably started your own library of pregnancy books and have signed up to a few pregnancy websites. The resources available for women are endless. If there is anything you want to know about pregnancy, birth or your baby a trip to the local library or Google is all you need do. What about resources for him?

Traditionally, quality resources for men have been very scarce. What is out there is either outdated or fails to really connect with men in a meaningful way. The lack of resources inspired us to create the *Being Dad* series of DVDs. What started out as a quest to see if other men were as hopeless as us quickly turned into a global odyssey to help dads in the US, the UK and Australia be better prepared for pregnancy, birth and beyond. While we have had the obligatory horror nappy change lessons, beer experts and financial tips, in truth making these films has opened up women's ideas about what their man is really thinking about the pregnancy and allowed the bloke to feel more at home about what he's going through. Through hundreds of hours of filming sessions (recorded mainly in pubs around the world . . . we're not stupid) we've learnt a great deal about what it means to be a man and a dad in today's world. We've also come to better understand how the relationship between a couple is affected during the journey of parenthood.

The role of fathers has changed quite a bit over the ages and differs substantially from culture to culture. It's not just the role of fathers that has changed; what it means to be a man has also changed.

The number one response from the dads we spoke to when asked what not to say to your partner during pregnancy and early parenthood was this: never say you feel tired. It's offensive to your partner, because she truly is tired. But when we dug deeper, what we discovered was a classic bloke idea—keep your thoughts to yourself and never let anyone know that you're struggling. And struggling they are. As many as 5 per cent of first-time dads get clinical depression after the birth of the baby. That's one in twenty. These are real, everyday, genuine blokes who have been caught off guard by the massive change in their life.

In days gone by the role of the Australian father was to be the breadwinner, the hunter and gatherer for the family. But times have changed. Today there are more women than ever in the workforce and our national obsession with property and a possession-rich lifestyle has seen a huge increase in double-income families. Men are no longer the sole breadwinner, and in many cases they are not the biggest breadwinner of the family. Then there's the increasing number of single-parent families. What does it mean to be a single dad?

It can be confusing to be a man in today's society. Are we supposed to be macho or a SNAG, buffed up or boyzone, hirsute or hairless, Jack Black or George Clooney, VB or Grange Hermitage? Depending on which edition of *New Weekly* and *WHO* magazine you read last, you can get it horribly wrong from one minute to the next.

Images of being a dad can also be very confusing. On one hand we see celebrity dads who are portrayed as cool. Sporting and movie stars who are snapped with their little ones after winning the grand final or cruising the Mediterranean between starring in billion-dollar blockbusters. Then there are the portrayals of the average dad as the bumbling fool who sticks a pin in the baby's derriere or puts on a nappy back to front. What are we? Cool guys or morons? Should we share centre stage with our wives or be shrinking violets in the background? How does one balance the roles of man, father and husband?

It's so tempting to listen to the moaning as we write: 'Stop whingeing . . . you've got it easy.' We're almost questioning writing this section. Why? We think it's actually fear that's at the heart of the problem.

Of course women have it tough. Way tougher than men. Not many blokes would swap places for all the beer in Germany, but that doesn't mean it's not tough on this side of the fence. In Ireland we heard an interesting metaphor. Let's say in a car accident a wife and a husband got injured. He broke one leg, she broke both legs. Both would go to hospital for treatment. They would both be allowed to cry out in pain and be looked after. Would you expect the hospital to treat only the wife, as she had two broken limbs? In a healthy society, would he ever stand outside the hospital not mentioning his injuries, as hers were much worse? Would the bloke be criticised for getting his leg attended to? As a society we continue to ignore men with broken legs during and after pregnancy. We aren't asking you not to think about your own issues; we're just asking you to also consider his.

Most guys today want to be a more involved dad than their own was. They want to share the responsibilities of parenting but they may need some assistance. Give him the right tools and resources, point him in the right direction and get him on the path to parenting. He has the turning circle of an ocean liner, so don't expect any radical changes overnight. It's a slow and steady change of course, but fortunately he has three trimesters to get it right—think of him as your tugboat into port.

In this chapter we are going to give him a heads up of what's happening to you and the baby in Trimester 1. We'll arm him with the basic information he needs and that will be of interest to him. We'll explain what morning sickness is all about, why he needs to be sympathetic and what he can do to help. So if you start seeing cups of tea and dry biscuits bedside in the morning you'll know who to thank, or blame.

Many guys have a hard time bonding with their baby in utero (in the womb) because they can't quite get that it's a real person in there. Most blokes, for example, describe the baby kicking the womb as like something out of the movie *Alien*. To get him up to speed on the development of your baby and make him realise it's a little person in there, we've procured a diary from a real baby who told us his story of life in the womb.

What's on his mind?

Nothing.

Yep, that's right, probably nothing. Zero, zilch, donut, nought . . . a golden duck. He's in complete denial still, despite the six positive pregnancy tests and a thumbs up from your doctor. Chances are he's filed all the facts under 'Do Not Disturb' or 'Pending', but we are planning on cracking through the thick varnish of denial and rubbing him back to reality. If we are successful, he'll start thinking about the following:

Money and finance, job security, mortgage payments

The psychologists tell us that money is his first worry because he can't see any tangible evidence that a baby exists yet. He will concentrate on tangible factors he can see, such as finance. The money issue is more about adjusting your lifestyle, and this actually seems to happen naturally. The over-the-top lifestyle naturally curbs itself, and the sheer volume of hand-me-downs and gifts from friends and family, along with the free on-tap baby food (your boobs), means that you're unlikely to shell out much cash for a while after the baby gets home. In time he'll understand that he isn't going to be destitute because you're having a baby, but it's a great idea to tackle the issue head on and work out a budget to put your minds at ease.

Did you know that in the old Western movies, the reason why the men were sent to get boiling water and blankets was purely to give them something to do? Blokes need problems to fix, answers to find, instruction manuals to ignore.

So let's learn something from John Wayne: it's a good idea to set him a task, with a timeline. Get him to sort out your wills, life insurance and health insurance. Use the time you have now to get your financial affairs in order. You could even organise a meeting with a financial planner. A good one can assist you with all the aspects of finance that you should consider now you have a baby on the way.

His space

For such small and sleepy things, babies require quite a bit of space. There is the cot, a stroller, the change table, the nappy bin, the chest of drawers, stuffed toys, more plastic Mattel crap than you can poke a stick at and God knows what else—it all starts invading your domain. You will want to banish all masculine accoutrements like golf clubs, bikes, surfboards to the shed. He won't understand that you need them out of sight in Week 8 of your pregnancy, which is when you go into nesting mode. Be kind: just despatch a few items a week until he realises that the only toy he has left in the house is a Matchbox car. Remember that he links his prized man possessions (regardless of whether or not he actually uses them) to his sense of self. Remove them too quickly and you may as well banish him to the shed. Which we seriously think you should not do. Slow and steady . . . no shocks to the system, please.

The car

For some reason, most pregnant women feel that it's not safe to transport a baby in a vehicle under 2 tonnes in weight without all wheel drive and a wheel base of at least 500 metres. Let's be honest: you want a 4WD that's capable of crossing the Sahara but will never actually get off the bitumen. It's the same reason we all go into the movies loaded with 4 kilograms of popcorn and 5 litres of soft drink—unnecessary but comforting. It's OK, really.

You need to have a very good battle plan for broaching the issue of a new car. Make a list:

1. why poo and vomit is easier to clean off leather than cloth trim;
2. how the laws of physics don't permit a stroller to fit into a sports car; and
3. how statistics say you and the baby would be safer in a Hummer than a Hyundai Getz.

Be prepared for a fight and avoid models that have sliding doors and more than six seats (such as the Toyota Tarago). You'll need to transition your cars as you add to the brood. By the time you've popped out number three he'll think the Tarago is a good bet, but right now he'd rather be seen in a 1962 Nissan Cedric with whitewall tyres.

Your relationship—is it strong enough?

Hopefully you have this one covered after Chapter 2. A good stocktake of where you are at and your expectations should have put his mind at ease. Let's take a deep breath, say 'Yes, we've done that', and move on. Truth be told, though, it's probably exactly that thought process that got you both in this mess in the first place.

The first ultrasound—why seeing really is believing

You've heard the saying that a picture is worth a thousand words. For most guys, this has never been more true than at the first ultrasound. Think about it: you've had physical and emotional changes, hormonal surges and a baby growing inside you, but he's had nothing other than watching you fall asleep at 8 pm every night.

Granted, the ultrasound pictures can be like a scratchy scene from the community TV channel that your antenna can't quite catch, but it doesn't really matter. For the first time he will actually believe that you have a baby on board. For many dads the first ultrasound can be very emotional. We've listened to dads from all around the world tell us how it made them get very sweaty eyeballs.

It's paramount that he comes with you to your first ultrasound. It's probably the most exciting part of the pregnancy experience for men.

Miscarriage

Miscarriage is a conspiracy of silence. No one wants to discuss it despite the fact that it's extremely common. Miscarriage is obviously enormously traumatic for women; it's a horrible experience for men too.

For many men it can take some months before they really believe or acknowledge that your bump is housing a real person. From the dads we've interviewed it seems that with an early stage miscarriage guys are most concerned with your wellbeing—their sense of loss is less. Guys are also likely to be more pragmatic about it, with a common view being, 'Well, at least we know we can get pregnant, we will be OK next time.' That of course provides little consolation for you.

Many women start attributing physical characteristics to their baby from very early on. No matter the size or stage of pregnancy, the baby is a real person with real features and maybe even a name. So for most women, a miscarriage is no different from the death of a family member or dear friend. It is a serious loss, and there is a grieving process. They wonder what they have done wrong, and feel that they have no one to turn to.

The partner's pain is in itself a heavy burden for the man. What to say? How to say it? How to acknowledge and manage his own feelings of loss? Many dads we interviewed discussed how difficult it was for them to deal with miscarriage—they felt they needed to be supportive of their partner and just did not deal with their own sense of grief and loss.

If you've being trying to get pregnant for a long time or if the pregnancy has progressed to a later stage, a miscarriage is likely to have an even more profound personal impact on both of you.

This is a delicate subject and we're only trying to show you that miscarriage will affect him too, and the effect could be as profound as it was on you. He will be grieving for himself and also wanting to help you with your sense of loss, with little idea of how to do either.

If you feel he is being unsupportive, or if he says the wrong things, it's not because he doesn't care. It comes back to his sense of helplessness and frustration that he can't fix the problem; he doesn't understand that you just want to talk about it and have him listen to you. Talking with friends and family about miscarriage can be helpful. You may be surprised how many people close to you have experienced the loss of miscarriage. Similarly, encourage him to talk to his friends. He may need to speak with someone other than you about his feelings.

It's also worth noting that if you have had a miscarriage, or several miscarriages, he may start getting very anxious when you fall pregnant. He'll be worried that you both may have to go through the experience again. It can be a very stressful time for couples and being unable to communicate and express how you both feel can make the situation much worse.

OK, now your work is done for the night and it's time to hand the book over to him. We are going to ease him into this pregnancy caper and give him one more relatively easy chapter to navigate before we start getting into the good stuff. Come the second trimester he'll be aware that changes really are afoot and we can start getting him up to speed on your changing and growing body. For now, though, we'll put a final focus on his favourite topic—himself.

FOR H♦M

Let's refocus on the situation at hand. You've managed to get your partner up the duff (whether you intended it or not), you've had a deep and meaningful about your relationship and what lies ahead and you're probably scratching your head wondering why things have started to change for the little lady without even a sign that there's a baby in the house:

- She's super tired and/or emotional.
- She's experiencing that old chestnut, morning sickness.
- She wants you to get her boxes of rubber bands to chew on or has developed a penchant for apples from the Lenswood region in South Australia.
- Your surfboard was relocated to the shed without your consent or knowledge.
- You came home and found her cleaning the shower grout with your Oral B toothbrush.
- She looks longingly at 4WDs and Toyota Taragos.

What about you? Have you started feeling anxious thinking about the future? Can you imagine what it's going to be like being a dad? From the moment you discover that you're going to be a father it's natural to experience a raft of emotions, from panic to elation and everything in between.

This is what dads we surveyed felt:

When you found out your wife/partner was pregnant did you feel ready to be a dad?

Yes	74.0%
No	26.0%

What was your major concern leading up to the birth?

Partner's health	57.9%
Baby's health	58.4%
Money	25.9%
Watching the birth	4.6%
Losing my social life	4.6%

Did you cry at the birth?

Yes	44.7%
No	55.3%

When the baby was delivered, what was your first emotion?

Joy	52.3%
Surprise	8.0%
Relief	37.2%
Love	29.6%
Other	11.1%

Do you feel less important to your partner than before the birth of your first baby?

Yes	32.0%
No	68.0%

Do you now think you were prepared to become a dad?

Yes	72.4%
No	27.6%

Here is a list of common concerns for guys in the first trimester.

Valid concern 1: Money

Money is one of the first things we all start thinking about. Will you need a bigger house? A new car? How will you survive on one income? How can you afford child care? The list is endless and can cause premature ageing, including baldness and grey hair.

The reality is that in most circumstances you just do manage. Naturally you adjust your lifestyle to fit around the baby and your levels of energy. You'll cut back on dining out, drinking and other areas of discretionary spending without even realising you're doing it. Talk to mates who have kids about how they adjusted.

There are several tasks you should complete in the next month, though. Doing them will put your mind at ease, impress your partner and reduce possible stress once the baby arrives:

1. Make a will together. Many couples don't consider a will until children are on the scene. Should the unforeseen happen, you'll want to make sure that your child is being looked after by a carer of your choice and that any money or assets are allocated appropriately.

    You can either get a will kit and do it yourself or do it with help from a lawyer.

2. Consider your level of insurance:

    - *Life insurance.* Ideally, insure yourself so that if something happens your partner and child would be provided for in terms of housing, income and education.

    - *Income protection insurance.* Your need for this will depend on your circumstances. Will you be a single-income family? What will happen if you fall ill or are unable to work?

    - *Health insurance.* Let's hope you have already changed your health insurance to a family friendly policy, or taken out such a policy. If you haven't done it yet, do it now. Kids get sick a lot, especially when they start socialising at day care or school. Often their ailments are contagious, so you can also expect to get your fair share of nasties.

3. Budget for the next year or two. The word 'budget' makes us shiver, and we'd rather lick the floors of a peep show

than sit down and do a budget, but it will save you a lot of worry and heartache. What extra expenses will you have, from health care to baby goods? How long will you be on a single income? Will you have a nanny or day care? If you're hopeless at finances get help from an adviser or friends and family.

4. Evaluate your financial style as a couple. The best way to tackle your money worries is head on, and the best time to do it is now.

Valid concern 2: Your space

Your house, duplex, semi, flat or caravan is about to shrink. For such small creatures kids require a lot of space, space that was formerly yours. Most of that space will be filled with completely useless crap that you don't need and will rarely use but will never be allowed to give away or throw out.

Baby clothes, cot, stroller, change table, drawers, more plastic crap than you can poke a stick at, 265 stuffed toys, mobiles, baby bottles, breast pumps, sterilisers, bouncers, porta-cots, nappy bags, baby carriers, car seats, play mats . . . it's goodbye to the spare bedroom or home office/gaming room.

Surfboards, golf clubs, expensive bikes you never use, dust-covered weight sets and all the toys that remind you of your youth may be headed for the garage. You'll want to fight it but it's a losing battle, so don't let it get you down!

Valid concern 3: Your car

If you have a sports car or a sensibly sized vehicle, chances are you will be discussing the safety features of Sherman tanks, 4WDs and vehicles with sliding doors. Where is the pram going to fit? Is it safe for the baby? Is there enough room in the back seat and boot? How do you get vomit off cloth trim? All reasonable questions that you'll be answering shortly.

That being said, sales guys have assured us that sometimes it's actually the guys pushing for the new, bigger car. So either way you may have a fight on your hands. Be prepared.

Valid concern 4: Your relationship

Is your relationship strong enough to make it? We discussed this in the previous chapter so we hope you've starting working on strengthening your relationship and enjoying your time together. If not, go directly to jail, do not pass go and do not collect $200.

What else can you do in Trimester 1?

The best things you can do for the next few weeks are:

1. Understand what is happening with your partner's body so you can be understanding, supportive and avoid saying/ doing things that will get you shot.
2. Start bonding with your baby by understanding what he is up to in the womb and how you can help build him through exercise and good nutrition.
3. Attend all doctor and ultrasound appointments.

Points one and two are covered in the next two chapters; point three is up to you.

The ultrasound—why seeing is believing

Attending the first ultrasound is an absolute must. Alongside your overpowering sense of denial, somewhere within you is the realisation that your partner is REALLY pregnant. If you're anything like most carriers of the Y chromosome you'll need physical evidence to help you believe that there is a baby inside your partner. Some say that the ultrasound was developed to help detect abnormalities with early-term babies, but the conspiracy theorists out there believe it was designed to prove to men that they are soon to be fathers. In truth, the ultrasound can effectively achieve both these things.

Dads from around the world have told us that the ultrasound picture is indeed worth a thousand words. It may make your chest pound or your eyes water, or it may just make you smile. It's your first look at your baby, proof that you're soon to be a dad and a very proud moment in your life. It's also pretty frightening.

At the risk of deterring you from attending, it can be scary. Everyone worries that they may not find a heartbeat or may detect another problem. Taking images from many angles means the physicians can look at everything from fingers and toes to major organs and blood vessels. They will also look for signs of Down's syndrome and other complications. Based on your partner's age, family history and the results of the scan you will be given a risk assessment for possible birth defects. Even great numbers like one in 35,000 can seem frighteningly small, and it's normal to be genuinely scared. Regardless, attendance is a must. In the vast majority of times it's to share in the amazement and excitement; in a very small minority it's to be there to support each other and to understand your options.

Many couples keep pregnancy a secret up until the results of the first ultrasound. There are pluses and minuses, of course; you get to enjoy the time to yourselves without being bombarded by friends and relatives, but if something does go wrong it tends to make you keep the secret, and that's not always healthy. At those times, you need the support of friends and family. One solution is to break your good news to those whose support you'd want if it went pear-shaped—your closest friends and family.

Physical changes

Even if it was a complete accident, you still have to marvel at the physiology involved in fertilisation. In Chapter 6 you'll read the 'Diary from the Womb' (page 117), which will give you an idea of what the baby gets up to over the nine months of pregnancy. What about your partner's body? What's happening physically and mentally over the nine months? Most importantly, how can you avoid the many pitfalls that have bought millions before you to their knees?

As we've discussed, blokes are by nature problem solvers and fixers. It's not really a problem unless you can fix it, right? Sure, sometimes she'll just want to complain and have you listen in silence, but where possible we will highlight issues you can help address.

We cannot profess to have even come close to understanding the intricacies of the female mind. We are getting better at listening, we understand the need for constant reaffirmation and we now know that we are always wrong, but that doesn't mean we are any closer to really understanding what transpires in the female subcortex. Unravel that mystery and you'll be up for a Pulitzer, a Nobel Peace Prize, a place in the Australian cricket team and an honorary Professorship in Psychology from the University of Dubbo.

We could have interviewed leading experts, actually asked a few women or gone to the library, but instead we used our favourite form of market research: pregnancy websites. As we discovered earlier, these sites are a hive of hormone-driven activity on which the spleens of the pregnant are vented by the thousand every second of the day. We've donned the Harry Potter cloak of invisibility, created a cyber persona and stalked the conversation boards for weeks on end to get to the bottom of the mysteries of pregnancy.

We've researched all the changes that will occur from fertilisation through to the end of Trimester 1 and reduced them into a fine jus for easy consumption. The following information will give you the ability to:

- Nod knowingly at doctor's appointments when terms such as 'perineum', 'episiotomy' and 'colostrum' are used.
- Feel comfortable to ask questions of doctors that won't result in a shake of his/her head and a death stare from the partner.
- Sound knowledgeable at dinner parties.
- Show the partner, mother-in-law and significant female others that you're taking an interest in the pregnancy.
- Save you from making relationship-ending comments to your partner.

Fasten your anatomical seatbelts, grab a low-calorie beverage and let's get stuck into Pregnancy Anatomy 101.

Week 1: Defcon 1

Most women don't suspect they are pregnant until they miss their period; even then most just think the train is running late. It's not until Week 6 that true signs of pregnancy start to arrive at the station.

Physical

The first signs of pregnancy may include slightly enlarged or tender breasts, a heightened sense of smell and a metallic taste in the mouth. The need to pee regularly and fatigue are also clearly apparent. So if she's sleeping on the toilet or says her breasts are sore she may be pregnant.

Mental

With fatigue will come the occasional mental explosion. If she normally suffers a bit pre-menstrually it may be completely undetectable, but if she's not prone to that you may get a sniff that something is awry.

Week 6: Defcon 2—nausea and morning sickness

Physical

Let's get one thing straight right now: morning sickness is real. It can occur any time of the day and is best described as like having a hangover for three months. Hats off to the ladies. A three-month, incurable hangover . . . We're just going to let you think about that for a minute.

Glad you're not having the baby! Morning sickness kicks in around Week 6 and can last for 6 weeks or longer. We've researched the caper to the nth degree in belief that it could possibly be complete rubbish, nothing more than an elaborate ruse against men. We've trawled through libraries, consulted microfiche files in medical institutions and bribed leading medical experts but are sorry to say we cannot offer you any evidence to refute the ailment and therefore stamp it as genuine.

No one has managed put their finger on the exact cause and there is no guaranteed cure, but many believe it is caused by digestive enzymes reacting to the HCG (human chorionic gonadotropin) pregnancy hormone. HCG is the stuff that is produced when the fertilised egg implants itself. Maybe it's just mother nature's bumper sticker that screams 'Baby on Board'.

Morning sickness is your first opportunity to help mum and baby. If she's experiencing morning sickness you can assist by giving her a cup of tea and some dry biscuits in the morning before she gets out of bed. Ginger is also thought to help ease morning sickness symptoms as is vitamin B6, which is in most pregnancy supplements and many foods including bananas and wheat.

Mental

If she's getting morning sickness it may range from unpleasant to debilitating. You can't fix it or make her feel better other than as suggested below. Offering some sympathy, and otherwise refraining from saying anything stupid or inflammatory like 'Keep it down in there, I'm trying to sleep' or 'It can't be that bad', is recommended.

All the pregnancy side effects and the raging torrent of hormones can create a Jekyll and Hyde–like persona. Here's a great piece of advice we picked up in our research: The smartest thing a man can do after winning an argument with his partner is apologise.

> **TIP 1**
>
> Nothing says 'I love you and I'm involved in this pregnancy' like a cup of tea and a dry biscuit every morning.

Constipation

Pregnancy is just an endless tsunami of hormones for your partner. One of the many hormonal side effects is constipation. Lots of water (2–3 litres) and lots of roughage (vegetables and fibre) are really the only natural remedies for constipation (other than reading on the toilet, obviously). We still don't get why women are disgusted by the concept of reading on the snapper lounge. We'll read anything from the back of a shampoo bottle to *Gone with the Wind* and we swear that's why we don't have any issues with the brown stuff . . . but we digress.

> **TIP 2**
>
> Buy her a paper each day . . . just kidding. Why not buy her
> an eco-friendly water bottle? Much healthier and cheaper
> than drinking from plastic bottles, and it makes it easier for
> her to keep track of how much water she's drinking each day.
> Not as romantic as diamonds, but there's nothing romantic
> about being egg-bound.

Weeks 6–9: Defcon 4—baby on board

Physical

Sometime between Weeks 6 and 9 you'll have done the test and
have had the thumbs up from a piece of plastic or a real doctor.
We've heard hilarious tales of guys who have made their partner
do the test kit half a dozen times because they don't believe the
result. Most of them because they are in denial, some because
they only had one nut and were delighted it was operational, and
some who even peed on the kits themselves to ensure a negative
result was in fact possible.

By now her breasts will be noticeably larger and her nipples
may be more prominent or darker. If you see small nodules
appearing around her nipples, make a casual passing comment
that she shouldn't worry, they are just Montgomery's tubercles and
completely normal. She'll be wowed by your blinding insight . . . as
long as you don't get them confused with the Mormon Tabernacle,
in which case you'll confirm your status as an idiot.

There is a good chance she may feel overwhelmingly tired in
the first trimester and you may be left to your own devices on
the couch after 9 pm most nights. Enjoy watching sports while
you can—her energy levels will return by Week 12 and you'll
be handing her tissues during re-runs of *Sex and the City* and
episodes of *Super Nanny*.

> **TIP 3**
>
> Keep her supplied with healthy snacks throughout the day to maintain her blood sugar levels and suggest that she should eat small meals regularly.

Mental

Just like you, she may start having some worries and concerns about being pregnant. Is she ready? Will she be a good mum? Will you abandon her? All that good stuff. It's important to keep the lines of communication open and regularly discuss how you're feeling. Lots of the normal worries and concerns can be eased by talking about them.

Other

We don't know whether pregnancy cravings are mental, physical or complete rubbish. Let's face it, given the opportunity to get away with eating any food you wanted because you have a pseudo-legitimate excuse, you would. Burgers, pizza, chocolate, the list goes on. It would seem that for some women it's just that—a great excuse to eat crap and not feel guilty. Can't say we blame them. Cravings can be for all sorts of stuff: sweet, salty, spicy and even healthy food like fruit. No one can explain the origins of cravings or if they are genuine. The jury is well and truly out on this one.

Just when you think you have put an end to the midnight craving runs in the middle of winter along comes the pica phenomenon, which creates a craving for non-food items such as . . . wait for it . . . wait for it . . . dirt, ashes, clay, chalk, ice, laundry starch, baking soda, soap, toothpaste, paint chips, plaster, wax, hair, coffee grounds, even cigarette butts. We met a guy whose partner craved boxes of new rubber bands, which she would smell and chew on!

Pica is the Latin name of a magpie, the bird that will eat anything—funnily enough, a bird also prone to attacking unsuspecting individuals when it has nippers in the nest!!

If it wasn't for pica we'd throw the book at pregnancy cravings. It's hard to argue that there's nothing to it when your partner is picking up cigarette butts off the street and chowing down on them. You'd probably rather kiss your partner after she'd eaten beer-battered pickles than a dirt and cigarette risotto.

What's the answer? If she has cravings, do your best to satisfy them. If they are unhealthy food items they are OK in moderation; if she's dressed in a Collingwood jumper and searching the house for rubber bands, put on a bike helmet in case she decides to swoop you!

Week 9: Defcon 3

Skin conditions

Hormones play havoc with her skin in early pregnancy and you'll probably have to listen to many rants about the state of affairs in this department. For some reason pregnant women start producing melanin, the stuff that makes your skin go darker in the sun. There is a phenomenon known as the mask of pregnancy, which describes the darker blotchy patches that appear on the face. Not as cool as the mask of Zorro or as funny as the movie *The Mask*, so just tell her she looks beautiful or glowing!

Talking of glowing, here is an interesting fact that you can pull out wherever appropriate: the term 'glowing', when used in pregnancy, comes from the fact that increased blood flow to the fine vessels beneath the skin on her face causes oils to be released from the skin's pores, giving it a shiny or glowing appearance. Completely useless fact but we bet you didn't know it . . . impress someone today.

Acne is also another major bugbear. Women prone to acne may get a breakout in early pregnancy. If she has it she'll be fully aware of it, so there's no need to draw attention to it. Once again, when asked tell her she's beautiful or glowing. Unfortunately, it doesn't stop there for the body's biggest organ, the skin, which can also experience tags, rashes, stretch marks, varicose veins and more. Fortunately for both of you, most of these will vanish once the baby appears.

TIP 4

Aim to say three positive things to her every day, starting immediately!

Bleeding gums

She may also complain of bleeding gums when she cleans her teeth. As you'll hear in the 'Diary from the Womb' (page 117), she's producing a lot more blood when she is pregnant. This increase in blood flow can cause capillaries (small veins) and soft tissue to rupture, making the nose and mouth prone to bleeding. A super romantic gesture is to buy her a soft toothbrush. We are all about the big ticket items here at *Being Dad*.

Week 11: Defcon 3—just Relaxin

Our favourite pregnancy hormone is Relaxin. Sounds like an R&B album by Usher but it is a real hormone. Relaxin's job is to help blood vessels stretch to accommodate the additional blood flow; the downside is that it can cause a drop in blood pressure, making the relaxin' one feel dizzy. Relaxin plays a few different roles; unfortunately, despite its promising name, it can't stop mood swings and irritability.

TIP 5

She will have the occasional emotional blowout and not so occasional bout of moodiness. Take it on the chin for what it is . . . the hormones talking. There's no point engaging, and no point inflaming the situation by reacting to it. Unlike UN troops, you may not engage with the enemy even when fired upon.

Miscarriage and complications

Miscarriage is very common. Contrary to popular belief, there is nothing you can do that will definitely result in a miscarriage. Miscarriage is normally a result of a chromosomal abnormality, and rarely means the loss of a healthy baby. Unfortunately, that doesn't diminish the sense of loss that comes with miscarriage. Miscarriage is often more difficult for women than men, but that doesn't mean it won't affect you.

It's important to remember that from the time she finds out there is a baby on board your partner is thinking of that little jelly bean as a real person, with human features and possibly even a name. It's a connection we fellas can only try to understand. As a result, an early-stage miscarriage is often far more devastating for women than for men. It's not uncommon for us guys to be unable to comprehend why our partner is so grief stricken when an early-stage miscarriage occurs. Our brains may be giving us logical instructions such as:

- At least you can get pregnant.
- You'll be OK next time.

- Miscarriage is common and a sign that everything wasn't OK with the baby, so it's not a bad thing.

None of these is likely to be any comfort to your partner.

While you may not feel an enormous sense of loss in an early-stage miscarriage, it will still affect you if your partner is grief stricken or has a hard time dealing with it. You'll want to help her, be there for her and make her feel better. However, there is little you can do other than offer a shoulder to cry on.

Loss in a later stage of pregnancy or after a long period of trying to get pregnant may have a more profound impact on you. As you start engaging with the baby and bonding with it you will feel that it is a real little person, just as your partner has felt from the very start. So you will have to deal with your own sense of loss, and you will also feel compelled to put your partner's wellbeing ahead of yours. Many guys have told us about the difficulty of dealing with both, about how they didn't voice their own grief as they tried to stay positive and supportive for their partner. If this happens to you and you feel like you need another outlet, talk to your mates who have had kids. You may be surprised at who else has had a similar experience and be able to get some good advice from them on how to deal with your loss.

Remember, pregnancy is the most natural human process and, like all natural processes, it isn't perfect.

*　　*　　*

That's a fairly sombre and heavy note to finish on. The first trimester really seems to just fly by. In some ways it's as if life hasn't changed much, but your baby is growing and you've probably started to detect some major changes in your partner. In the next chapter we'll look at those changes, how you can cope with them and how you can start bonding with your baby.

Chapter 4
Sex during pregnancy

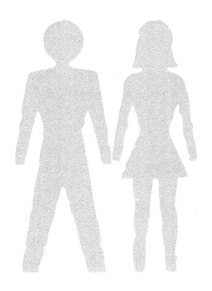

FOR H♀R

Sex during pregnancy is a topic that needs a great deal of consideration, exploration and debate. If there is one thought in that vacuous mind of his, it's sex. He's a man, so he's capable of thinking about sex during a funeral, a football game or dinner at your parents' house. It's not as if he can control the sex part of his brain . . . it's been poorly wired by evolution and nothing is likely to change that.

If there is ever a time in your relationship where your sexual timetables clash it's going to be the next 12 months. Like two out-of-control trains travelling aimlessly on the London Underground, you may not ever arrive at the same terminal at the same time unless you get to the control panel and start fiddling with the levers.

We've spent way too much time surfing the community boards of pregnancy websites undercover as a pregnant woman, trying to get to the bottom of where you girls lie on the issue of sex during pregnancy.

We don't think there is a definitive answer as to whether women have an increased or decreased sexual appetite through pregnancy. It would seem that there are periods of 'Don't come near me' and periods of 'I'm a raging nymphomaniac', with relatively calm times in between.

We're not qualified or stupid enough to try and coach women through their sexuality issues but we can help out when it comes to your man, whether you need to keep him at bay but happy when you're not interested or get him on the job when you're dying for it.

On one online survey we saw, 12 per cent of women said they wanted more sex than they were getting and 27 per cent said they'd rather stab their man than have sex with him. Well, that's not entirely true; the 27 per cent really said they just had no interest in sex. We're not sure what happened to the remaining 61 per cent—they must have been off having sex or stabbing their husbands.

Let's explore the complex sexual issues that arise during pregnancy so that you can enjoy your celibacy in peace or orgasm to your heart's content.

Is he a can or a cannot?

We've interviewed hundreds of men around the world for our *Being Dad* films and it doesn't matter what colour, religion or nationality they are, all blokes fit into one of two categories:

1. Sex during pregnancy offers no issues and they are bang up for it, as always.
2. While still finding their partner sexy, they lose their mojo.

So is your man a can or a cannot? What can you do if your sex drives aren't in sync? How can you penetrate his grey matter to pull in the reins or re-ignite his mojo?

The sex talk is a conversation that should take place before you get pregnant or in very early pregnancy. We know it's a hard thing to discuss, but sex and intimacy are important parts of your relationship and a change in them can cause emotional issues for both of you unless you can communicate on the subject.

We know you don't want to hear this and we'll probably get slammed for bringing it up, but a surprising number of men and women are unfaithful during pregnancy because of differing sex drives. It's the truth, so let's have a good look at problems and resolutions.

The can do man

Who's a lucky girl then? Or are you?

The can do man is up for it day or night right up to the birth, which is fabulous if you actually have a sex drive but a nightmare if sex is the last thing on your mind. Don Juan or sexual pest . . . it's a fine line. If you're not feeling sexual during pregnancy, what are the reasons? Is it a short-term thing or has it been going on throughout your pregnancy?

Too tired, feeling unwell, not feeling comfortable with your new body, he's an annoying slob and you'd rather torture him than pleasure him, worried about the baby, it's painful? These are just a few of the reasons that our fellow November birth club BFFs told us. We were also told that some women's sex drive fluctuates between trimesters, some want it all the time and some just have zero desire for the whole nine months.

How's a bloke to know whether you're up for it—and if not, why not—unless you talk openly about it? Sex, as you know it, will change for the next few years. You'll have less time, be more tired and will genuinely despise each other for short periods of time. Sounds sexy, doesn't it?

Here are a few good reasons to get organised (have sex) while pregnant:

- The increased blood flow to your nether regions can result in things feeling pretty good down there and orgasms can be simply mind blowing! (Or so we're told.)

- Pregnancy brings a great opportunity to re-invent your sex life. For many couples who have been together for some time frequency may have dropped off or it may have become as predictable as the Christmas sales. Logistically, you need to explore new positions to find what works and what doesn't and it can also be a great time to re-introduce foreplay and other non-intercourse forms of sexual interaction if they have been on vacation.

- This is the last time you'll be just the two of you for at least 18 years. Try to enjoy it!

Explore the possible reasons for not feeling into sex and ask yourself, 'Can we fix it?'

- He's not making you feel sexy—get him to read this chapter or organise a hot date (preferably with him). Buy some new sexy undies and a new dress or top. Look sexy and you may feel sexy.

- Sex is painful—experiment with lubrication and mix it up with some extended foreplay. As the advertisements say, see your doctor if pain persists.

- He's an annoying slob—trade him in or hire a gigolo (just kidding!). Explain to him that if he helped out more you wouldn't be so tired and grumpy and that may lead you to feeling more inclined to have sex.

- You don't like your new body—we're yet to meet a man who didn't describe his pregnant partner as beautiful. Who wouldn't want to explore your new body?

If, after reading the inspirational piece above, you're still unable or have no desire to have sex, you need to tell him why. Will you get upset if he masturbates or looks at pornography? Chances are he'll be doing one or both if he has an extended period of celibacy.

If he's doing something wrong, let him know. If it's something completely unrelated to him, explain the problem. If he's pouting and thinking that this is the beginning of the end, you may have problems soon.

Communication is the key. As long as he knows your reasons and how you feel, chances are he will be understanding.

The can't do man

If a guy tells his partner he isn't interested in sex or can't do it during pregnancy she often suspects that he just doesn't find her attractive any more. It's not true, so don't believe it.

Most guys think their partner is very sexy while pregnant. Pregnant women look fabulous and the extra curves are fun, so what are the real and legitimate reasons for some men struggling with sex during pregnancy, particularly late-stage pregnancy?

- He's scared of tapping the baby on the head.
- He feels as if someone else is in the room.
- It's a girl.
- Logistics.
- He's scared of hurting you.
- He thinks that his semen may induce birth.
- He doesn't know that your orgasms could be earth-shattering.
- He's forgotten that being intimate need not be just about intercourse.

You'll be pleased to know we've explained exactly why he doesn't need to worry about these later on in his section on page 89. You're welcome, ladies!

Sex is healthy for your relationship and the baby, and it's bloody good fun—or it should be! If you're really struggling to get him across the line, ask your doctor to reassure him that sex during pregnancy is good for all concerned.

The tendency for blokes is to either pout if they are not getting enough or withdraw if they are feeling sexually insecure. If you're mindful or each other's fears and concerns and open about your feelings, your ying and his yang should get in sync.

Hand over the book to your man now. When he's finished reading this section will be the best time to talk sex, then have sex, then talk some more about sex.

FOR H*M

Sex during pregnancy is a topic that needs a great deal of consideration, exploration and debate. What does pregnancy mean for your sex life? Is she going to be a raging nymphomaniac or a nun? What about you—what can you expect from yourself now that she's expecting?

Do pregnant women get horny?

Pregnancy and birth are characterised by myths, wives' tales, conspiracies of silence and bald-faced lies. We're sure you've heard that at some point in pregnancy women turn into insatiable sex machines. You might think sex will induce labour or be scared of tapping the baby on the head.

In this chapter we will bust some myths, put the ruler through a few wives' tales and tell you why even if your partner does turn into a nympho it might be you that gets the yips. Let's start at the beginning. What does happen to a woman's sex drive during pregnancy?

We didn't want to waste time in the microfiche section at the state library looking up old research reports on the subject. Frankly, we couldn't care less what generation A was doing way back when our grannies were promiscuous or what the hippies in the 1970s were up to when under the influence of hallucinogens. What about today's sexually liberated generation W, X and Y.

So where could we go to find such information? MySpace died, Facebook's dying and Twitter just annoys the crap out of us so we went back to the parenting boards on the leading parenting websites. We know we've mentioned these sites before, but we implore you to get on them yourself and read what women just like your partner are talking about on them. It's more fun than Guitar Hero, more educational than the History Channel and it's free.

While researching the topic of sex (it's a tough job) and trawling through posts on babies' names, best baby wraps, ultrasound visits and the like we found an entire conversation with over 380 responses on the following topic: 'Which is the best anal lubricant?' Some of the posts would have made a sailor blush. It all came complete with a survey, and one of the options was dog saliva! What was even more disturbing were the results of the poll. See below . . . this is legitimate.

Which is the best anal lubricant?	
Dog saliva	14 per cent
KY	36 per cent
Vaseline	2 per cent
Olive oil	2 per cent
Other	46 per cent

Source: http://community.babycenter.com/post/a10470785/best_anal_lubricant

Crumbs. What has the world come to? We'd not even heard of brands like Easy Glide, Innuendo and Anal-ease, which made up the 46 per cent of 'Other', but they all sound a lot more pleasant and hygienic than dog saliva. We thought it took half a bottle of tequila and a bit of luck to gain a backstage pass. We just had to share that one with you . . . we're not sure if we have a point here, but if we do it's that pregnant women and new mums are online right now talking about how they want it and you don't, or you want it and they don't.

We've spent hundreds of hours on these types of boards, posing as fully fledged members of the uterus-carrying club, and have gained more insights into the female mind than we'd anticipated or hoped for. Unfortunately, when it comes to sex drive during pregnancy we've come to the conclusion that there is no guarantee your partner will be a nymphomaniac, and if she does when it will happen. What we can tell you is the following:

- If she's not feeling into sex and you're bugging her about it, expect to see your name up in lights on a pregnancy forum.

- Most women seem to have periods of heightened sexual desire and periods of zero interest at some stage in their pregnancy.

- Many women report that orgasms during pregnancy are the best they have ever had.

- Helping out around the house and telling her she is beautiful increases your chance of having sex by 1000 per cent.

Interested to know more? Read on . . .

If you work for the Bureau of Meteorology or you're a bona fide mad scientist we suggest you get into the shed and start tinkering with designs for a sexual barometer. Instead of your standard barometer that predicts useless things like rain, sunshine and humidity, how about inventing a sexometer that gauges a pregnant woman's daily sexual desire—which, from all accounts, is as unpredictable as the weather itself. Maybe that's what Doc Kegel (we'll meet him later) was up to when he devised the vaginal air pressure machine . . . we knew he was on to something.

Imagine the delights of looking up from your bowl of Weet-Bix and gazing at the sexometer to see that the little lady has swung from 'Never having sex again' to 'God, I'm dying for it' overnight. It would certainly make life a hell of a lot easier, although there may be a heavy body count during the testing phase of the device.

Riches await the inventor; it would certainly be an iPhone app with a difference.

Sexometers aside, what can you do if she wants it but you don't or you want it but she doesn't? (We're hoping you can work out the middle part of this Venn diagram for yourself.) How do you avoid being knifed, and how do you keep the nymph at bay if you're not so keen to play?

We hear plenty about women's sex drive during pregnancy, but very little is made of the fact that guys can also suffer from performance issues or lack of interest.

Are you a can or a cannot?

We've interviewed hundreds of blokes and it doesn't matter what colour, religion or nationality you are, blokes fit into one of two categories:

1. Bang up for it as always, big belly and all.
2. Suffer a loss of mojo once the baby starts showing.

What will you be: a can or a cannot? What can you do if you and your partner's sexual timetables conflict?

The sex talk is a conversation that should take place before you get pregnant or in very early pregnancy. We know it's a hard thing to discuss, but sex and intimacy are important parts of your relationship and a change in them can cause emotional issues for both of you unless you can communicate on the subject.

It's not uncommon for men with expecting wives to be unfaithful. They aren't getting it at home so they look elsewhere. You may feel disconnected and distant from your partner and may start worrying about your future in the sex department. Talking about it all will make you feel better, and may help you discover a solution.

The can do man

The problem with being a can do man is that you're keen to have sex all the way through pregnancy but there are likely to be times when she isn't. What's a man to do then? Keep your pencil in your pants, and refrain from pouting for starters.

Here is a legitimate list of reasons she may not be feeling like sex and some suggestions to remedy them:

- *She's too tired.* This is particularly common in the first trimester, but occurs throughout the pregnancy. Are you doing your part around the house? Are you making sure she's getting enough rest and letting her sleep in on the weekends? The more you do around the house, the more rested and relaxed she is, the greater the chance she will feel in the mood.

- *She's feeling unwell.* Morning sickness, heartburn, constipation, sore back, cramps, incontinence, flushing, piles, to name just a few possibilities. When she's not feeling brilliant she's hardly going to be busting to get it on. Be patient. Wait for the sexometer to swing back in your favour and help its movement by being understanding and supportive.

- *She's not feeling comfortable with her new body.* You might love her new boobs and curves but she may hate them. Compliment her regularly—try to say three positive things to her every day. If you make her feel sexy and beautiful she's more likely to want to jump your bones. If she was an exercise-aholic before pregnancy she may be depressed at not being able to work out hard. Do what you can to keep fit together: walk, pregnancy yoga or whatever helps her get the endorphins mobile again.

- *She hates you.* We know 'hate' is a strong word, but those hormones are strong. At some point she's going to hate your guts for a trivial slip up like getting drunk, coming home late, eating a food that makes her nauseous or looking like the bloke who got her in this state in the first place. You wouldn't poke a hornet's nest, so take a few deep breaths and wait for the pendulum to swing back again. There is nothing you can do here, pal, so move on.

- *She's worried about the baby.* Sex is good for everyone, including the baby. Hormones produced during sex and orgasms are thought to be positive. Get her to talk to your doctor. Also reassure her that you will be careful about putting weight on her belly and breasts and that you will be gentle. Start out slow, pretend you're fifteen again and see how much pleasure you can both get from fooling around without actually having penetrative sex.

- *It's painful.* Don't be afraid to try lubricants or spend some extra time getting her in the mood. Be slow, and be gentle. If it's still painful for her, ask her to talk to her doctor.

These are just a few of the reasons women list for not feeling up for sex.

How's a bloke to know whether she's up for it—and if not, why not—unless you talk about sex openly? It's a bit like fishing: you need to be patient, and be prepared to wait through long periods of sometimes inclement weather until the fish come on the bite. When they do, go for it.

There's no point whingeing, pouting or being overbearing. Help out, reassure her she's beautiful and that you love her and make sure she's well rested. Be understanding when she's not in the mood and make the most of it when she is. Most importantly, be open and communicate how you're feeling. We know . . . it's unnatural!

The can't do man

The can't do man can be left feeling completely emasculated. Let's face it, how often have you turned down sex with a woman who is desperate for you? It's hard enough trying to come to terms with what's going on with you without also having to deal with the emotional blitzkrieg from her. On the whole, pregnant women despise you for turning them down for sex. They are so used to you wanting it all the time that a refusal to engage can be seen as a hostile act: 'Why would you not want to have sex with me? Is it because I'm pregnant? Do you think I'm fat? Don't you find me attractive any more?' It's an emotional minefield that is likely to cost you an appendage or two unless handled with care.

First of all, if you're a can't do man don't feel bad; you're not alone. You're not even in the minority. Most guys we interviewed confessed to issues in the nest during pregnancy. The biggest problem is that they can't talk to their partner about the problem, because she straight away makes an incorrect assumption and the apple cart is turned over.

The can't do man, in most instances, still finds his partner attractive, even sexy, but there is some legitimate issue that kills his mojo. Let's have a look at the most common reasons why the can't do man can't do it.

- *You're scared of tapping the baby on the head.* It is amazing, but true, that some guys still believe it's possible. Here is the ugly truth, lads. In order to reach the baby you need to get through the cervix. We don't care how big you think you are . . . you are not that big. Second, during pregnancy a mucous plug is formed at the entrance of the cervix to protect the baby from infections and other nasties, including you. If you're really worried about it talk to your doctor or try non-penetrative sex.
- *You feel as if someone else is in the room.* If it was Jessica Simpson you probably wouldn't be complaining but when it's your child it's understandable. This is probably the most common reason guys give for just not being able to go there. You can combat this feeling with oral and other non-penetrative forms of sex, using positions where the bump isn't so visible (behind or on

your side), trying a vibrator until you get used to the idea of fooling around in the baby zone or just turning the lights off.

- *It's a girl.* Many guys who knew they were having a girl said that it made them feel very awkward to be getting intimate with their daughter so close by. In essence it's the same issue as the point above so we'd suggest the same options.

- *Logistics.* It can be a nightmare to find the position that gives you access and makes her comfortable. You may need to spend some time working out how to best tackle the problem. It's a great opportunity to explore some new positions, so try to have some fun with it.

- *You're scared of hurting her.* Communication is the key here, plus understanding what's OK and what's not—not putting too much weight on her stomach or breasts, for instance. Work out what the best positions are, how much force you can use, whether lubrication is required etc. Also, if you have lots of cushions and pillows around, it might help make you feel she's comfortable and protected.

- *You're worried your semen may induce birth.* Semen does contain prostaglandins that can kick start labour. It's not likely to have an effect much before the due date, though, so you're not likely to have to perform a home birth minutes after you've got down and dirty. Be prepared—if your partner is overdue she'll do anything to speed up labour, including DEMANDING you have sex with her. As you will learn, even when labour starts you'll have plenty of time to get to the hospital or check the PH in the birthing pool.

- *You didn't know her orgasms could be HUGE.* It's possible that female orgasms can be intensified in late-stage pregnancy due to the general swelling and increased blood flow to the nether regions. Don't tell us you wouldn't like to lock in the best orgasm of her life.

• *Being intimate need not be just about intercourse.* There are plenty of ways you can play around without having intercourse . . . maybe you need to go back to the drawing board. Many of the problems with a lack of intimacy can be addressed through communication. Sex is healthy for your relationship and for the baby—and let's not forget, it's bloody good fun! The tendency for blokes is to pout if they are not getting enough or withdraw if they are feeling sexually insecure. You need to be mindful or each other's fears and concerns and open about your feelings; that will give your yang and her ying the best chance to get in sync.

*   *   *

Bear this in mind: sex as you know it will change for the next few years. You'll have less time, be more tired and generally despise each other for periods of time.

So try to work through your issues together now. There are many reasons for not getting around to having sex during and after pregnancy and it's an easy habit to get out of. Make the time, use pregnancy as a way to reinvent your sex life and talk openly about how you'll stay on the job after the baby arrives.

Chapter 5

Trimester 2

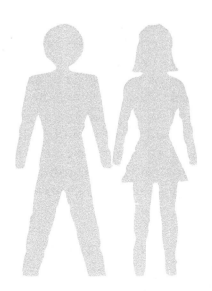

FOR H♀R

We're hoping you've broached the big issues that arose in Trimester 1 and his surfboard is keeping your new 4WD company in the garage and his playroom is now a lovely shade of baby blue.

As you traverse the trimesters and your body continues to transform you'll be having hormonal surges and a myriad of physical complaints. You're no longer you—well, you are you, just not the you he knew before you got pregnant, thanks to you know who . . .

Baby brain, nesting, cravings, swollen bits, big or bigger boobs, moodiness, skin breakouts, wildly fluctuating sexual desire—it's as if you've been possessed. In some ways you have: that baby is generating some serious hormonal activity that you can't control.

This transformation will not be going unnoticed by DH. He's probably come to realise that when he gets home tonight he may be dining with Dr Jekyll or Mrs Hyde. Take a step back from the nausea, constipation, fatigue and swelling and give a few moments' thought to that lovable bastard who got you in this position. What's going on in his mind this trimester? How can you keep him on course? What do you need him to be doing for you?

In the next few months the following issues are likely to enter his grey matter.

The in-laws

You've broken the news to all and sundry and now parental influence is starting to exert itself. If you're having the first grandchild, the relatives are probably hovering like vultures and he will be realising that their presence is going to increase exponentially in the future. They will be keeping a close eye on him to make sure he's pulling his weight and will be quick to identify any unacceptable behaviour now that he's going to be the father of their grandchild. The pressure is on.

How do you get along with each other's parents? If they live close by, how often will they be dropping by once the baby is born? It's time to discuss these things and set ground rules that are fair and equitable for all sides of the family. In-laws, yours and his, can be angels or devils, so if you foresee any issues tackle them head on now.

It's not just your parents that you need to consider. Let's face it, in some ways everyone's family is weird. Babies seem to bring out the weirdness and it's not always the good kind of weird. Favouritism, jealousy and general tension can surface. Patch up any unresolved issues and try to have your relationship with everyone headed in the right direction. These people are potential babysitters now, people who will allow you to glimpse the life you once led. It's time to kiss and make up, clear the air and schedule them in for one Saturday night a month!

Weight gain—yours and his

Some guidelines for pregnancy weight gain are issued by the US Institute of Medicine, most recently in May 2009. You're probably clued in to this, but we've included the stats in his section later on so that he knows what's going on.

But you may be wondering if guys really care about your weight gain? The answer to this is—honestly—no. As long as your weight gain is healthy and you're not endangering your health or your baby's, most guys don't really think too much about it. That isn't to say it's not a cause of many a dispute.

Thanks to all those ludicrous celebrity-laden magazines, there is a preposterous expectation that all women look like supermodels when they are pregnant and will shed the baby weight as quickly and easily as Madonna sheds a style. That expectation is, in our opinion, held by women and not men. We appreciate that you're going to get bigger and we are petrified of what it will do to your mental state.

'Does my bum look bigger?' is a question that will strike fear into the heart of any man. He wants to answer that question, and any question relating to your weight, in the following way: 'Yes, of course your bloody arse looks bigger—it is! You're having a baby and that's part of the deal, but you look fabulous and I'm loving the curves and bigger boobs. You'll be back to normal in a few months, so just relax. I love you.'

But of course he's way too scared or emotionally crippled to actually say that. He is more likely to blurt out something that will cause World War III for a few days.

Eat in as healthy a way as you can (which he can help with) and exercise. Revel in being pregnant and know that all men think you're hot. Even if he's a can't do man, it's not because you're bigger; it's because there's a baby in the room.

When it comes to his weight many blokes 'go out in sympathy'. They eat more and exercise less. It takes a joint effort to stay healthy during pregnancy and it will make birth and beyond more enjoyable and manageable. We discuss nutrition and exercise in Chapter 6. In the meantime, go and check out your bigger butt and boobs in the mirror. Revel in it—you look hot. Now go and grab your man and have a spontaneous and wild sexual encounter in the kitchen.

Phew! We bet that made you feel better! Back to business . . .

Sex—will he ever get any again?

Go girl! You're all over this. If you've just solved this probing issue in the kitchen 10 minutes ago he probably doesn't know what hit him, but we'll bet he's pretty happy with himself (and you).

If you ignored our advice and omitted the kitchen sex fest he's probably moping about the garden, listening to sport on the ABC and wondering if his and your best days of sex are past. Of course they aren't, but sex during pregnancy can't be a guessing game or no game; not talking about your sexual desire, or lack of it, can and will cause issues.

You may well be worried about the same thing. As the great Ron Barassi once screamed at his team of charges during an AFL grand final, 'Don't think: do.' Problem solved. Thanks, Ron. If in doubt, go back and re-read the previous chapter.

Responsibility—can he handle it?

Will he be a good dad? Will he be a good husband? How will he juggle the work/life/marriage balancing act? Chances are you have asked the same questions yourself. He may seem to be cruising through this pregnancy caper, but deep down in his subconscious a war is raging and at some point it's bound to surface. Our advice is to reinforce to him throughout the pregnancy that he will be a great dad. Get him to talk about what he feels would make him a 'good dad' and anything he foresees that would make him not able to meet his and your expectations.

As we asked early on: do his expectations of what a good father and partner are meet yours? What are the differences, and how big are they? They may seem small now, but when Cyclone Bambino hits town even small weaknesses will get exposed. Batten down the hatches, plug the leaks and tie down loose objects.

Your ailments

Because we love you, in this chapter we are going to give him a blow-by-blow account of all the ailments you may experience from here on in. We will list them, legitimise them and convince him that they are real.

Our aim here isn't to embarrass you—it's to make him sympathetic to the cause and get him helping you and the baby. Read through the following section for him and feel free to quiz him to make sure he actually took the time to read this important stuff.

Your baby-catching dream team

We've included some pointers on page 107 to help hubby choose the baby-catching team, which you might be interested in reading too.

FOR HIM

Okey dokey, lads, this chapter is a lesson in female anatomy. We'll skip the part on the female reproductive system, as it would seem you have already familiarised yourself with that piece of kit.

We've spent months interviewing the best medical minds in the western world and out of frustration we even consulted some ancient types in the far east, but we can't find any evidence to prove our hypothesis that the following ailments are really just a figment of the pregnant woman's imagination. So it is with great regret that we include the following as genuine ailments that you'll have to cope with, support her through and attempt to remedy.

For those shameless enough to not think this is important, we say skip this section at your peril. The end of the chapter focuses on you and your needs so be sure to at least read that, you selfish, egocentric Neanderthal.

It's all about her—and don't you forget it.

Being an expectant father is like being the invisible man without the upside. Most of the time you're completely ignored . . . but you still can't walk into the women's change rooms at the gym without being arrested.

Whether you're at a dinner party, the doctor's office, having an ultrasound or walking through Woolies, if you're with a pregnant woman it's the same deal. No one cares to think, let alone ask, how you're feeling about becoming a dad, how the baby is doing or when it's due. Most of the time you may not notice or care but there will be times when being the third wheel can really piss you off.

The alternative isn't much better, we guess. Imagine you had a whopping great beer gut that was brewing golden, frothy ale due for bottling in nine months. You'd probably get tired of old blokes telling you to look after yourself and the grog, your mates and strangers wanting to touch your stomach lovingly and people not standing for you on the bus when you're desperate for a seat. We digress . . .

Accept that you're the third wheel. However, there is no need to be a shrinking violet at the important times—at the doctor's or when drunk at dinner parties. So how can you actively participate in the social and medical aspects of expectancy? How can you look knowledgeable and interested and feel capable of intelligent contribution?

You may have no real desire or need to discuss the baby or the pregnancy, but appearing engaged and interested does make your partner feel that you want to have the baby and that you won't be a complete disaster at the birth or at parenting in general.

Unfortunately the only logical way you can achieve this is by having some idea what is happening with your baby's development and your partner's body. Pick up a pregnancy book for women and you can get a very comprehensive run-down on the minute-by-minute changes in every body part from the cerebellum to the cervix. For most of us it's information overload.

Fasten your anatomical seatbelts, grab a low-calorie beverage and let's get stuck into the next section of Pregnancy Anatomy 101.

Physical changes

Week 14

Achy Breaky Heart

Heartburn is a bitch. We know because we've suffered from it and our hearts goes out to women on this one. Our heartburn is usually self-inflicted and expensive, caused by over-indulgence in alcohol and rich food. We feel sorry for ourselves but it's hard to get sympathy from others. For pregnant women, however, it's all due to the 'moaning whores' again.

A slackening of the muscles at the entrance to the stomach can allow stomach acid to rise up, causing a very uncomfortable and at times painful sensation. Later in pregnancy it can be caused by the baby pushing everything north.

What can you do? Keep her away from acidic things such as fruit juice and spicy things such as her favourite vindaloo. Milk and yoghurt are good, and if she's really suffering she should speak to her doctor about suitable over the counter or prescription medication.

Does my bum look big?

Simple answer to that is no. In truth, yes, most things are getting bigger, but as we know it's for a very good reason. Do not look at pictures of pregnant movie stars and ask, 'Why don't you look like that?' Weight gain is normal and healthy.

There's no real way to successfully get out of the question 'Does my bum look big?' It's like having a shotgun pointed at your face and being asked if you'd prefer one barrel or two: it's going to hurt either way.

What you'd love to be able to say is, simply, 'Yes! It does, because it is bigger,' or perhaps, 'Darling, yes, your arse is bigger but it's OK, you're carrying a baby and it's supposed to be bigger. You'll bounce back to your normal size once you've had the baby and besides I think you look gorgeous—me lurves the big boobs!'

We recommend you don't say either of those despite the fact they are the truth and perfectly logical. Tell her she's beautiful and/or gorgeous frequently and try to head off the 'Does my bum look big?' train at the pass.

TIP 1

If she's complaining of heartburn, remind her to stay away from spicy and acid food and beverages. If she's complaining about you non-stop, send her to the day spa while you sneak in a game of golf.

Week 17

Physical

We're quoting this directly from WebMD.com because it made us laugh:

> You may notice an increase in vaginal discharge, or experience nasal congestion due to an increase in fluid levels. On a more positive note, these pregnancy hormones can add lustre to your hair and a glow to your skin.

We don't know about you, but we couldn't give a shit what our hair was doing if our vaginas were discharging all over the shop . . . We'd be staying in until said discharge abated. Once again, it's time to take a moment and reflect on the benefits of being a man and remember that there isn't much glory in being pregnant. Other than the fact she's growing a baby and has a lustrous new bonse, the whole caper sounds pretty miserable . . . and she's only up to Week 17!

Week 18

Captain Flexible

Surging hormones are causing ligaments and muscles to stretch more than normal. The upside is greater flexibility but the downside is increased risk of injury because of the additional weight she is carrying. Backaches and other body aches are common.

If you have a bath at home try running her a bath a few times a week with some good old bubbles and a trashy magazine.

> ### TIP 2
>
> Buy some heat packs, ice packs and some comfy new pillows. You'll be able to use them during the birth as a natural pain reliever and administering them during pregnancy is a sure-fire brownie point gainer.

Week 21

Captain Colostrum

Question: Can milk be released by the breasts before birth?
Answer: Yes, it can. A straw-coloured liquid called colostrum may start leaking from her nipples. This can happen as early as the middle trimester and can be sporadic. She may need to start wearing bra pads, so be sensitive. How would you feel if you had incontinent nipples?

> ### TIP 3
>
> If you're having sex and she starts leaking, stay cool and let her know a bit of colostrum isn't going to get in your way.

Cramps

All the extra weight being carried around is putting strain and stress on muscles in the stomach, back, bum and legs. Throw in girlie bit cramping that can range from mild to severe and all of a sudden pregnancy really sucks. Cramping and pain that don't go away can be a sign of problems, so if she's complaining for a few hours it's worth suggesting calling your doctor.

Exercise, good nutrition and lots of water may help.

Week 29: Not strictly Trimester 2, we know, but . . .

Squashed organs

The growing baby places a great deal of pressure on many of her organs like the liver, stomach, intestines and bladder as well as the diaphragm. She's feeling bigger on the outside and squished on the inside, so she's in need of your lovin' . . . of the emotional kind.

Hey, who farted?

According to an article we read on Babycenter.com, the average punter produces between 1 and 3 pints (600–1800 millilitres) of gas each day and passes wind about fourteen times a day. We're staggered that farts are measured in pints! We're not sure how to convert that into middies, schooners or pots . . .

During pregnancy gas production rises significantly. We don't think you'll be able to connect your partner to the BBQ or water heater, but you may need to keep the windows open or put the pet budgie outside.

Funnily enough, one of the main reasons she's producing more wind is an increase in progesterone levels. Progesterone slows down digestion, causing more gas. Later in pregnancy the abdominal cavity is a full house, causing even more pressure on the stomach and slowing digestion even further.

*   *   *

So there you have it: a very basic list of just some of the problems and pains she will experience. And now, to help her with all these problems, here is a shopping list for you:

- soft toothbrush
- eco-friendly water bottle
- dry biscuits
- tea (whatever her favourite is)
- some man pills for when she gets moody
- heat and cool packs
- new pillows and a pregnancy pillow
- a subscription to Foxtel (education and entertainment plus it has 24 hour kids' channels . . . and a fashion channel . . .).

Mental changes

There is a phenomenon known as baby brain that can occur in the first or third trimester. There hasn't been any testing done that proves women are actually suffering from a cognitive relapse when pregnant, so it may just be that there is so much going on in their minds there is no room left to remember where they put the car keys, to get milk on the way home from work or that you were supposed to be playing golf on the weekend. Let's face it, we blokes suffer from all of the above even when we have nothing on our mind or in our womb. A cute gift idea is to buy her a baby brain diary so she can write daily lists of what she needs to remember and do.

When you think about what's actually occurring inside her, which you will learn in the 'Diary from the Womb' (page 117), it's clear that there is a hell of a lot going on. It's complete anatomical chaos, so it's no wonder she's prone to moments of complete insanity, rage, hatred, forgetfulness and every other emotion known to man. It's easy to be annoyed, frustrated, angry or hurt by the outbursts (not farts) but they will pass (farts may not). The best thing you can do is help out, be supportive and take the king hits on the chin . . . God speed!

'What about me? It isn't fair, I've had enough now I want my share'

What about you indeed? Chances are you have had enough already, and you're nowhere near the finish line. Well, our friend, Trimester 2 is likely to bring about a few mental and physical issues for you too. Here are a few common ones.

The in-laws—you're going to be seeing a LOT of them

If you live in the same solar system as your in-laws, let alone the same street, suburb, state or country, chances are you'll be seeing a lot more of them (and your parents too, for that matter). How do you get along with them now? How will you feel about them being around a lot more often, dispensing useless advice?

One of the best things you can do is sit down with your partner and talk about who can come over and how often. If you have a patchy relationship with either set of parents, try to mend it quick smart. Babies raise lots of issues within families, and just like your relationship with your partner it's best to lay some ground rules, discuss expectations and generally strengthen family bonds.

Remember that family will soon become a very important source of babysitting, which will allow you back onto the streets, into restaurants and pubs and the real world again, so be kind.

Her weight and yours

We all know that when it comes to women, any question that involves weight is a tricky one. With the sea of raging hormones she is experiencing, this issue can become even more difficult to deal with. Generally, guys are fine with their partner putting on baby weight. We understand it's part of the process and that they can and will return to normal. Trashy women's magazines are always displaying model types who seem not to add as much as a nanogram while up the duff and within minutes of delivery are back to bantam weight division. This crap can put unrealistic expectations into women's minds.

If you really care about weight or are worried that she is eating poorly or gaining an unhealthy amount of weight, there is something you can do about it: exercise and diet. Walk with her, cook her tasty and nutritious meals and be sure to do the right thing yourself. Read Chapter 11 on building a baby for detailed information and tips on cooking and exercising.

Healthy weight gain—hers, and yours!

Some guidelines for pregnancy weight gain put together by dieticians were issued by the Queensland Government (see www. health.qld.gov.au/nutrition/resources/antenatal_wght.pdf), most recently in August 2009. Here are their recommendations:

- If her pre-pregnancy weight was in the healthy range for her height (a BMI of 18.5 to 24.9), she should gain between 11.5 to 18 kilograms, gaining 400 grams per week in the second and third trimesters.

- If she was underweight for her height at conception (a BMI below 18.5), she should gain 12.5 to 18 kilograms, or 500 grams per week in the second and third trimesters.

- If she was overweight for her height (a BMI of 25 to 29.9), she should gain 7 to 11.5 kilograms. If she was obese (a BMI of 30 or higher), she should gain between 5 and 9 kilograms.

- If you're having twins, she should gain 16 to 24 kilograms if she started at a healthy weight, 14 to 23 kilograms if she was overweight, and 11 to 19 kilograms if she was obese.
- All women can expect to put one or two kilograms in the first trimester.

Putting on excessive weight can be dangerous for mum and the baby and can lead to complications and gestational diabetes.

What about your weight?

Plenty of guys 'go out in sympathy' during pregnancy. Keep up (or start) your exercise program and make an effort to eat well and get plenty of rest. Being fit really helps during the birth and the first few months of being a dad!

Are you ready to be a dad?

It's normal to worry about your ability to be a good dad and partner. You can ease these worries by writing down what you think constitutes being a good dad and partner. Ask her to do the same and then work on making your expectations align. Also, try to work out what barriers in your current life might stop you becoming the type of dad you'd like to be and how you can work together to overcome them.

Choosing your birth team

If you're like most blokes we've interviewed over the years you probably think that when it comes to choosing your birth team your partner knows best, so you let her be a one-woman selection panel. Yes, it's true, women generally do know best . . . and even if you don't believe that it's often best to acknowledge it when in the presence of a pregnant woman. That said, you're going to be working closely with this team of people to deliver your baby so it's important you know who they are, what they will do and that you can get along with them. Why not get involved in the process of choosing the team? You're probably an expert at who should be playing for the Australian Test XI or pulling on the jersey for your favourite football team, so why not employ those skills in this most vital decision?

Don't sit on the sideline. There is no fantasy league for this sport—get involved with the selection process, because your birth experience will be much better if you're around people you get along with and have confidence in.

Does it really matter who helps deliver your baby? Absolutely! Think carefully about it. Choose together. People who can help catch your baby include: obstetricians, hospital midwives, birth centre midwives or homebirth midwives (or even you—preferably with the guidance of a trained professional). Talk to people about their medical providers and interview a few different people. You'll probably be surprised at what you learn.

Obstetricians are doctors who specialise in gynaecological and obstetric surgery and vaginal birth. They are trained to care for higher-risk mothers so some say they are trained to look for problems as opposed to trusting the birth process, but that depends on the doctor's experience and personality. Obstetricians can and do also care for low-risk mums. Meet with them, ask them questions and try to get to know them. Don't be afraid to shop around.

Family doctors (GPs) can catch babies when mum and baby are healthy and labour is going well. Midwives approach birth as a healthy and normal event while monitoring mum and encouraging her body to do what it was designed to do: give birth. Midwives work in a variety of settings: homes, hospitals and birth centres.

If you don't ask questions you'll look like a goat, or uninterested, or both. Here is a list of questions that will make you sound and look knowledgeable and help you pick the perfect baby-catching team:

- What is their philosophy about birth?
- Do they encourage their patients to get epidurals?
- How do they feel about (and what is their experience with) unmedicated birth?
- How do they feel about birth doulas? A birth doula is a person trained and experienced in childbirth who provides continuous physical, emotional and informational support to the mother (and father!) before, during and just after childbirth. The word 'doula' comes from ancient Greek, meaning 'woman's servant'. So in some respects you can also consider yourself a doula of sorts.
- Who else is in their practice and do they share the same philosophy about birth?

Most doctors and midwives do not deliver babies every day of the week. They have designated days each week that they are at the hospital or birth centre, and they will care for patients who are in labour on those days. It's possible you could have someone at your birth who you've never met.

Ask them about their statistics: What percentage of births they are involved with are induced, or receive epidurals, or are Caesarean deliveries? How long do they spend with mums in labour? How many babies have they delivered? . . . and anything else you're curious about, such as can they run 100 m in under 12 seconds and which football team do they follow?

As well as picking who will help you with the birth, the two of you also need to decide where you would like to have the baby. Your options include a hospital, birth centre, at home or in the car park in Woolies (hopefully not!).

Write the following questions down in a book, take them along to the meeting and wow your partner with your interest and preparation.

Questions for a hospital

- Will you both feel comfortable there?
- If there's a choice, what are the differences between the hospitals in your area?
- Are there different possible models of care at the hospital?
- How does that hospital's Caesarean birth rate compare with the rates of others in your area?
- Are there showers or bathtubs in any of the labour rooms?
- Do they have birth balls?
- What is their policy on taking pictures and videos?
- Is an epidural available at all times?
- Are there monitors that allow mum to walk down the hall and around in her labour room?
- What kind of nursery do they have? Some hospitals can care for very small or very ill babies; others need to transfer those babies to another hospital.
- Do they provide childbirth classes? If yes, also consider out-of-hospital classes as an option.
- How can you schedule a tour?
- Is there always a lactation consultant there during the day?
- Do they have a rooming-in policy so that babies aren't separated from their parents?

Questions for a birth centre

- Will you feel comfortable there?
- How far is the birth centre from a hospital?
- How do they determine who gets transferred to a hospital?
- Are there tubs or showers in every birthing room?
- Where do they recommend you take childbirth classes?
- Do they provide doulas or do you bring your own?
- Do they have birth balls, squat bars, etc.?
- How can you schedule a tour?
- Is the midwife with you at all times during labour?
- How long do you stay there after the birth before you go home?
- Does someone from the birth centre come to visit you at home?

Questions for the manager at the local supermarket

- How often do you clean the car park?
- How far to the local hospital and what are the directions?
- Do you have a mobile phone and can you call 000?
- Do you know how to deliver a baby?
- If we have the baby here and it makes the news, can we have a year's worth of nappies for free?

*   *   *

As you will no doubt have identified, things are really starting to heat up. You want to enjoy the experience of birth and make the first few months of being a parent as stress free as possible—the more you do and learn now the better. Your partner will really start to slow down soon, so you need to start helping out, getting involved and being supportive. By helping her you're helping your baby.

Soon we'll check in on the baby and see what's going on in there. You'll marvel at just how amazing the development has been to date and what's yet to happen. We'll explain how doing dishes results in more sex and start preparing you for the big day.

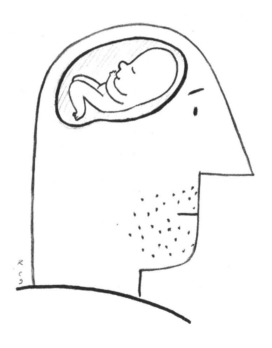

Chapter 6

Bonding with the baby

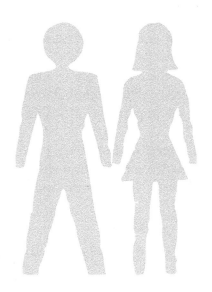

FOR H♦R

In just a few chapters we've come so far. We hope that by now we've averted his course towards the river DeNial and steered him in the direction of acceptance. We've told him that he is going to be a dad, talked with him about how your relationship will change and discussed expectations. He has some idea of what is happening with your body and will soon learn about the amazing development of the baby week by week. That's a good start, but we still have many months to go and much work to do.

The next step in the evolution of dude to dad is getting him bonding with the baby. We have read dozens of books on pregnancy, birth and parenting; you can imagine the looks we get on the treadmill at the gym as we flick through the classics like *Baby Love*, *A History of Birth*, *Feeding the Bump* and *The Natural Way to Better Birth and Bonding*. All these books are fabulous resources that are brimming with great information, but none gives much real estate to men and the importance of bonding with the baby in utero.

We've given this bonding caper a great deal of thought and have come to the conclusion that we need to consider the workings of the male mind to solve the problem. In order to process information effectively we blokes need:

- evidence that something exists (tangibility)
- identification of a problem that could require our skills to solve or fix
- a good reason to be bothered to work on said problem
- positive feedback that we are on the right track, and
- an outcome in a fairly short period of time.

We can use the same process for pregnancy and bonding with the baby:

- Step 1: Prove a baby exists—ultrasounds, grow a belly, complaints of unusual ailments and cravings.
- Step 2: Make him understand that the baby needs help to grow and that he can play a role through nutrition, exercise and making your life easier.
- Step 3: Demonstrate how his efforts will help develop a healthy baby (rave about his healthy cooking and how it makes you and the baby feel great).
- Step 4: Use further signs of growth, such as baby movement and foetal feedback, naming the baby and talking/interacting with it.
- Step 5: Being there to help with the birth.

Boil it down and what we're really getting at is that in order to bond with his baby your bloke needs to feel like an integral part of the process, a co-driver in the Bathurst 1000 and not a spectator drinking beer on the top of Mount Panorama. The key ingredients to this are:

- attending the ultrasounds and doctor appointments
- getting into the kitchen and cooking food for you and the baby
- exercising with you
- coming up with a nickname for the baby and starting to interact through talking and music, and
- understanding how he can help you (and his baby) at birth.

We've already given him the heads up on the ultrasound, so in this chapter we are going to teach him a thing or two about nutrition and exercise. Does he know how to cook? If not, consider signing up for some fun cooking classes. They are a great date and could pay big dividends in the years to come. Encourage him to get in the kitchen now.

These days there are plenty of blokes who are at least as good in the kitchen as their partners (or better!). Even if your man does know how to cook, knowing what foods are responsible for growing a brain, muscles, bones etc. will give him an extra sense of achievement when he dishes up your next meal. We are about to show him how he can 'build a baby' through nutrition.

Bonding with the baby seems to take longer for guys, so getting him on the right path now is worthwhile.

Let's get on with the bonding . . . and cooking . . . and exercising. The next chapter for him includes 'Diary from the Womb', which is a blog written by a real baby that explains the week by week changes. You might like to read it; after all, it's your body he's talking about.

FOR HIM

In this chapter we are going to explore how to start bonding with your baby while he is in utero. To do that we need a good understanding of what he's up to in there and how we can have a positive influence on his growth, development and wellbeing.

Bonding with the baby can take us a while, so it pays to get a head start by interacting with him now. It's not hard and it can be a lot of fun; it's like a science experiment that actually means something.

In order to give you a good understanding of exactly what your baby gets up to in the womb we asked a sperm to write a blog about his experience of the journey from the testes to the womb and beyond. It's a real account and a novel way for you to follow your baby's growth and development.

Diary from the womb

31 December

10 pm, pre-launch, inside the testes

Dear Diary,

Word filtered down from the brains trust that we should prepare for evacuation. We've been put on code RED—this is what we've been training for. Intel reports suggest that the target egg was seen leaving its ovarian location at 1600 hours today.

The two-week boot camp in the epididymus was tough. Motility training was a bitch and millions of blokes didn't make the muster. Last week I passed the final training requirements and was moved up to the Vas Deferens, where we await deployment. Seventy-four days of swimming training and seminars about what lies ahead has taken its toll on many. Over half of my fellow recruits are a mess and stand no chance of making it as far as the cervix, let alone the egg.

It's pretty crowded in here, with about 200 million of us ready to go over the top. Only one of us will live to fight another day, assuming a successful fertilisation. I'm feeling super fit and ready to go. My swim coach, Field Marshall Thorpe, says if I can get a good lane and don't do a false start I'm a great chance to make it to the egg first. He's always so positive, and he still holds the record for ball to egg 80-centimetre dash—he's a spermatazoan god.

Lately we've been hearing horror stories about deployments that have gone wrong. Several of the last waves of men have ended up flailing in underpants or swimming aimlessly for days on bed sheets due to poor co-ordinates being used on live firing. Life must have been so much less stressful before SpermTube and other sperm networking media—it's so easy to take bad news on board these days.

5 January

6 am, Week 3

What a journey! Battle stations were manned at 12.05 am and the artillery was positioned for firing. I managed to squeeze into lane 4 in the left teste as per Thorpedo's instructions, but there wasn't much warning when the big bang finally happened. Two hundred million of us shot through the urethra and into a hot LZ (landing zone). To say it was chaotic is an understatement. Men were falling all around me, some were swimming in the wrong direction due to shell shock and many went down due to the acidity of the hostile environment. I was mid-pack as we traversed the cervix and by the time we hit the Fallopian tubes there were only a few thousand of us left in the charge. Faced with a decision as to which tube to take I flipped a coin—tails left, heads right. Tails it was.

By the time I finally made it to the egg I was sure my days were numbered. There were three other sperm already there trying to gain access. I noticed two of them had funny-shaped heads and just couldn't get through, and the third, Trevor from my graduating class, was just too exhausted and was dozing with his head on his tail. I just tucked my tail in tight, made a beeline for a vacant spot and went straight through—I couldn't believe it.

Once inside things started happening pretty quickly. I exchanged genetic details with the ovum immediately and once all 46 chromosomes were accounted for I headed off for the RV (rendezvous point).

Spent the next three days dividing into more and more cells and travelling down the fallopian tubes towards the uterus where the plan was to dig in (implant) to get vital resupply of nutrients from the hostess. Once I reached the endometrium (lining of the uterus) I deployed the necessary hormones to allow me to settle in and await further instructions.

It was a very emotional journey through the Fallopian tubes. I saw thousands of dead and dying comrades—all that training just to die in the heat of battle seems like such a waste of youth. Many cheered me on with the last wag of their fatigued tail. It bought a tear to each of my sixteen cells.

On a positive note, I have some Big News: I was promoted today from the rank of Private Sperm to Corporal Zygote. If only Mum and Dad could have been here, they'd have been so proud.

19 January

Week 5

Seems the mission is progressing well. After successful attachment to the uterine wall I've started taking on blood and nutrients and am feeling much better. Another promotion, this time to the rank of blastocyst: Sergeant Blastocyst (sounds menacing, I know).

I've started producing my own hormones now so I'm hoping the host will soon be notified that my mission has been successful and she'll stop drinking that awful cask wine . . . it tastes terrible even after filtration and cleaning.

I have deployed the vending machine (placenta) which will transfer fluids between me and the hostess. This appears to be working already and I'm undergoing considerable internal changes every day.

28 January

Week 6

Well, the hostess seems to be providing some pretty funky nutrients. I'm growing like crazy and I've started looking like a tadpole again.

I seem to have developed a heart, and if I don't mind saying so myself, I'm massive. Weighed myself on the scales today and couldn't believe my non-existent eyes. I've stepped up from microgram weight division into the gram division and I'm a staggering 3 centimetres long—it must be all the vitamins and minerals I'm receiving from the accommodating hostess! She even seems to have stopped drinking that awful wine and I'm not detecting any nicotine, which is good, as it was giving me wild head spins.

Unlike the early days back in the testicles, I'm not doing any tough training sessions to get stronger and bigger. I'm simply bludging by the side of the uterus all day, drinking and piling on the milligrams . . . they didn't tell us the mission would be so easy!

It would appear that I have a very big head and tiny heart—just like my dad!!

28 February

Week 10

Changes are afoot—literally. Well, I don't know if it's a foot yet, but I've developed four stumps that feel like they will be arms and legs. Looks like my tail is about to fall off and the best news is I'm growing eyes! Can't wait to check myself out . . . hope there are some reflective surfaces in this joint. I feel a million times bigger than when I was in sperm training.

It's getting a bit boring in here so I'm going to try to move around a bit and see what I can find. Without a tail or legs I'm not sure how I will manage.

It's amazing the changes within. Without even knowing how, I've developed a stomach, liver and a few other vital organs. Checked my pulse my ticker is doing 150 beats per minute and I'm not even sweating. There's no doubt about me—I'm miraculous.

Wrote to Mum and Dad today to let them know I've been promoted . . . AGAIN! I now hold the rank of Warrant Officer Foetus. It doesn't sound as exotic as Zygote or as menacing as Blastocyst, but a promotion is a promotion. Note to self: must get new business cards printed.

The vending machine is doing a great job. I connected the supply hoses as instructed in the manual and it's like an all-you-can-eat buffet 24/7. What a great design—now I can float about freely and still get a feed. As an added bonus, every time I think I need to do a pee it just seems to go back up the tube and into the vending machine . . . brilliant. Whoever designed this set-up thought of everything!

28 March

Week 14

Things just keep getting better. I've started growing a brain . . . well, if I could think, I think I'd think it's a brain. I'm still struggling with this sudoku book I smuggled out of the testes but things seem to be happening upstairs. Speaking of stairs, there seems to be a new annexe under construction downstairs as well. If only I had hands . . . I could get down there for a feel and see what's going on.

Strange devices have started growing on the side of my head and they are talking to me. I keep hearing strange sounds. Last week I had a weird sensation, as if someone was taking pictures of me—I could feel unusual sound waves travelling through my body and it felt as if someone was staring at me! I covered my southern annexe with one arm and stuck up my other fist to whoever it was trying to perve on me.

At the same time my host was sending weird messages I couldn't decipher—tears of joy at seeing me, or something like that. I have also started noticing a deep-voiced unit that is regularly attached to the hostess.

In other developments, I'm getting teeth and have now started breathing and swallowing the fluid I'm suspended in. The first few mouthfuls were bloody awful but I got accustomed to it soon enough. There are all sorts of new things growing inside of me. I have no idea what they are supposed to do.

Jumped on the scales again today and they went right off the Richter scale. Bugger me . . . I'm another weight division up since I last checked. Seriously, I'm one huge mother's foetus.

28 April

Week 18

Have started calling these things on the end of my arms hands, because they are very handy! I can't stop touching myself—I feel awesome. Re the downstairs issue, there's something sticking out down there. I will be interested to see it one of these days. I wonder what it's for? Maybe it's just a toy to play with when I get bored.

Arms seem to be getting longer, which is definitely helping with my dance moves. For some reason, when the host is moving around I just want to close my eyelids and have a kip but when she's still I'm ready to party and bust some serious moves. I seem to be able to contort my face into different shapes, which is really helping my dancing.

The pool seems to be getting bigger, which is lucky, as I'm still piling on the weight. Also piling on some sort of fuzz on the exterior. It's not a great look but it's keeping me warm when I'm not disco dancing.

I'm weighing in at about 180 grams and am 13 centimetres long. I amaze me.

28 May

Week 22

OK, what's going on? I'm dancing like a mad man trying to keep the grams at bay but it seems the more I do the fatter I get. I'm going to have man boobs and serious back meat if this continues. I was a whopping 260 grams a few weeks ago and I've been way too anxious to get on the scales since. So much for eating right and exercising! I'm dancing, stretching, flexing and doing everything I can with the limited resources in here. I hope I'll start bulking up soon—am keen to get buff.

Those things on the side of my head are definitely talking to me now. I can hear music, which makes me want to dance. I'm particularly fond of the music the one with the deep voice keeps playing. 'Ice Ice Baby' by Vanilla Ice and 'I'm Too Sexy' by Right Said Fred are wicked tracks and really get me moving.

The fuzzy stuff is now covering my head as well as the rest of my body—what the f+ck is happening in here? I've been trying to communicate with the vending machine to change my diet to make this stuff stop growing. I'm careful not to upset it, though, as it continues to transport my wee out of the pool. What sort of animal would urinate where it has to swim?

Crap . . . just hopped off the scales: 450 grams. I'm as fat as a house.

28 June

Week 26

Today I had my first thought. I was just dancing around minding my own business when my brain started communicating with me. It wants to know when we are getting out of here . . . I didn't know what to tell it. I think it's broken . . . I can't switch it off. It keeps sending me messages. Stupid brain . . . what do I need it for anyway? I've got everything I need already. Plenty of food and drink, nice house, arms and legs that let me dance. I sense this brain will get me into trouble one day. Maybe I can learn to not use it.

Weight check: 560 grams. I'm a glass half full type of foetus but I'm now closer to a kilogram than a gram, and it seems like yesterday I was microscopic . . . where is my life going? Do I need to start thinking about my future? Damn brain—shut up!!!

The one with the deep voice keeps talking to me. He makes me laugh—calls me all types of stupid names, like Wamey and Tiger. Doesn't he know my name is Eugene? That's what the hostess keeps calling me. While I'm on the hostess, she continues to be fabulous to me. I don't know what I'd do without her . . . I take her for granted too much. Maybe I'll try not to push up against her bladder so much tonight.

14 July

Week 28

I've stepped up the diary entries as there is so much going on. My brain just won't shut up. Keeps saying things like $E=mc^2$ and that in the case of a right-angled triangle A squared plus B squared equals C squared, where C is the hypotenuse. What the f+ck am I supposed to do with that information? I certainly don't require it when doing what brings me the most joy—dancing and touching myself south of the umbilical cord (that's what my brain told me the tube to the vending machine or placenta is). All these new words and thoughts . . . I just wish I could go back to being a zygote, when I didn't have a thought or worry in the world.

On non-brain related news it seems my march toward the kilo weight division means I'm running out of room in here. Need another annexe built on quick smart. Had to do a three point turn the other day to change direction.

My body now has a delightful white substance covering it. I know this because I can open my eyes, see light and generally scope things out.

PS I'm a very good sort.

28 July

Week 30

The hostess is always moving around and fidgeting. Doesn't she know that I need some rest? It's getting very cramped in here and I'm no Kate Moss. Smashed through the 1-kilogram barrier last week.

I'm seriously considering getting out of here and having a word to the hostess.

The deep-voiced one keeps prodding me and telling me to give him a kick. He'll get a kick all right, right up the arse, when I get out of here. The hostess has been complaining that he's a lazy sod who is in for a real shock when the baby comes. Don't know what that means but it sounds as if he's in for a tough time—he deserves it.

I've been peeing a lot and I don't think it's all getting removed as efficiently as I'd like. I'm now swimming and drinking it. No wonder I've started getting the hiccups! Body hair starting to fall out, fat addition showing no sign of abating. Brain keeping me awake at night and I'm getting bored with the view. Might see if I can break out of here somehow. Have started booting the walls, which gets a reaction from the hostess but doesn't achieve much else.

14 August

Week 32

Still can't find an escape route. It's getting bloody tight in here and I'm spending most of my day just thinking about stuff and trying to work out what's going on on the other side of the walls. My new brain helped finish off the last of the sudoku book so I'm literally just twiddling my thumbs.

There have been lots of people trying to touch me. The invasion of privacy is outrageous. They're prodding me night and day—the nerve!

For some reason I keep wanting to lie upside down. Some strange force within is telling me to do so. I can't work out whether it's my brain, the hostess or the vending machine trying to issue the instructions. I get the feeling something is about to happen. I've been going over my evacuation notes from sperm school just in case.

My brain keeps on getting bigger and better. I'm able to control it better and I think I'm learning how to do things. For example, if I want the hostess to sit still I just apply pressure in certain places and hey presto she stops moving.

Weight check: here cometh 2 kilograms.

28 August

Week 34

My eyesight is getting better and I can see things much more clearly. I can now distinguish between night and day—have requested some sunglasses from the quartermaster but they are yet to arrive.

Am still fascinated by the arm between my legs. It looks lovely too. I've developed a thick white coating on the outside of my skin that's not sexy at all. At this rate I'll be single forever—that's what my brain told me, but I have no idea what it's talking about. Seems the only time my brain stops working is when I touch my leg arm. How curious.

I'm officially out of room in here and am having to spend a lot of time stretching and trying to get comfortable. Sometimes I get fed up with the lack of space and give the hostess a good old boot.

Sucked on my thumb today—who's a clever foetus then?

14 September

Week 36

Ouch . . . scratched myself today with my fingernails and it hurt. Might give the hostess a scratch and see what happens. Maybe I can scratch my way out of here . . . I feel like my time in here has come to an end. It's getting claustrophobic, boring and I feel I'm as well developed as I'm ever going to be. I've had enough of this fluid as well, it's starting to taste terrible. I suspect I'm drinking my own wee in large volumes—not happy, Jan. I've also noticed that the food coming from the vending machine is starting to taste different. Last night something came through that was super spicy.

I also seem to have something gathering inside me that I have an urge to dispel. Something is telling me to wait because the placenta can't get rid of it and whatever it is isn't going to smell or taste brilliant. I have a strange desire to read.

28 September

Week 38

Yesterday the vending machine issued a new mission to me via my brain. Seems I can't do anything these days without my brain getting involved. The mission reads:

Evacuation imminent STOP Rest up STOP About face and engage head into pelvis at stage 5 STOP Await ripening of cervix to 10-cm dilation STOP Commence forward push through birth canal STOP Exit vagina STOP Await further instructions STOP Godspeed OUT

As much as I love military speak, I have no idea what any of this means but my brain is now running the show. Since the instructions arrived I've positioned myself upside down in the engaged position. I'm trying to relax and conserve energy, because I sense that the days ahead could be physically demanding and I'm well out of shape.

I've noticed that I now have eyelashes, and that leg arm has got much bigger in the last few days. Pity it is so crowded in here— having a hard time finding the space to play with it.

1 October

Awoke this morning to an eerie gurgling noise and watched in horror as the pool I've been swimming in for the last nine months started emptying. At least I now know where I'm headed. The walls around me have started squeezing regularly, pushing me towards the opening. It's getting bigger slowly and I can see the light! I'm a little scared about what lies ahead and what the future may bring.

2 October

WOOOW. What a day. So much has changed since my last journal
entry. After the water emptied from my swimming pool and the
exit door started opening the walls started squeezing harder and
more frequently, pushing me forward. As per the mission instructions
I waited for the doors to be 10 centimetres open before really starting
the forward offensive. Talk about tight! I thought I was cramped for
space in the uterus. The birth canal was so tight I could feel my head
getting squashed and I had to do a great deal of wiggling my hips
and shoulders to shimmy forwards.

All the while the hostess was making a lot of noise . . . the deep-
voiced one was very quiet. After a long time, when I was sure I was
stuck, my head started sliding under and up through the pelvis. The
first sign of departure was a very cold feeling on the top of my head.
I felt very panicked and a bit distressed but the training from sperm
school came back and I relaxed and concentrated on the job at
hand. It was a lot of hard work manipulating my head and shoulders
to navigate the tight space. There was no turning back from here and
all my concerns disappeared as I surged forward.

The pushing of the walls was driving me forward, and just when
I least expected it I was pulled from the safety of my home and
into a brave new world. Fortunately, the vending machine was still
attached and sending me air and other supplies—like a good wing
man he stuck by me the entire time. Once outside I started to breathe
in a foreign substance that was much easier to suck in than the pool
water. It filled my lungs and made me feel fabulous.

What really shocked me was the size of the beasts handling me. I
thought I was huge, but these guys were ENORMOUS. I was placed
onto the hostess—she felt warm and lovely and when I looked into
her eyes it was the most beautiful thing I'd ever seen. She's dreamy.
She also has two big soft pillows with suction ports that looked very
inviting. The vending machine, which was left behind, was still
sending me messages from the battle field, and it told me to storm
the suction ports and latch on for dear life . . . which I duly did. As I

latched on I watched as one of the white giants gently pulled on the supply cord, helping the vending machine from the battle field. We were together again . . . or so I thought.

Shockingly, one of the white giants clamped the supply cord, cutting off communication, and handed the deep-voiced one a threatening silver device. Deep voice then severed the tube . . . from within I let out a mighty roar, screaming for them to stop, but the vending machine sent one last communication telling me his job was done and that I needed to go on without him. He told me to stay close to the hostess and the deep-voiced one and to latch on to the suction cups when hungry or scared. With that he was carried away and I'm yet to see him again. I'll make that deep-voiced one pay for the rest of my life.

I'm exhausted from the mission and am needing a long sleep. The suction ports don't seem to be giving me much food as yet . . . I hope the vending machine knew what he was talking about . . .

Nutrition—how you can build your baby, bond with your baby and save your marriage!

Now that you understand just what happens to your baby week by week, it's easier to work out how you can help with all that amazing development. In researching this book we've read dozens and dozens of books on pregnancy, birth and parenting, so many we're in danger of growing a uterus via osmosis. What has stood out to us are two things:

1. They are as exciting to a man as a bamboo skewer inserted through your testicles; and
2. They offer very little advice for what dads can do to help bond with the baby in utero (the womb, that is).

As we were removing the latest bamboo skewers from our gonads it struck us that we blokes can play a very important role in the development of our babies and at the same time bond with them in utero.

We're Australia's un-handiest men, so blokes like Tom the Chippy and Jamie Durie shit us to tears (yes, we're jealous of them for their looks and skill sets), but the prospect of building something from scratch still appeals to our manly instincts. Nine months is a long time to wait for your baby. Would you like to help build him and in the process maybe bond with him before he's ready to emerge?

The following chapter is here not because we want you to know all this stuff on nutrition, but because we want your baby to be healthy, we want you to start bonding with him now and this will all help you look brilliant . . . three valid reasons to battle on.

Why finesse around for months putting the cot together and still get it wrong when you can be in the kitchen building your baby? Yep, you read us right. You can actually be responsible for building your baby. In order to reach all the development milestones you just read about, he needs the right tools—they come in the form of nutrients, and that means . . . food.

If you could pop down to Target, pick a baby making kit off the shelf and spend the next nine months building ears, a nervous system, muscles and a brain for your future kid and there was no risk of completely ballsing it up, it would be a pretty good way to spend the next few months . . . while your partner complains of nausea, swollen ankles and constipation. 'Darling,' you could say, 'don't interrupt me. I'm building Shane's spinal column right now. He'll need that to bowl ripping leg breaks and unplayable wrong 'uns . . . we'll worry about painting the nursery later.' Alas, you can't do any of this.

You can't choose the sex, hair colour or height of your baby— that happens at fertilisation. But from the time the zygote implants itself into the uterus you can start the building project. You can take responsibility, in part, for building essential items like a brain, heart, nervous system, teeth, muscles and strong bones—all the important stuff a person needs to play footy or be a ballerina.

The female anatomy is an amazing piece of kit that can perform some truly incredible feats when it comes to baby making, but it needs fuel and this is where you come in. By helping ensure that the fuel she puts in her tank is the highest quality you can assist with the performance of your little one. You wouldn't put ethanol in a Ferrari, so why put crap fuel into your growing baby?

Your baby is what its mother eats and drinks. Just about everything good and bad that passes her lips makes its way into him. He can only use the fuel that she takes on board leading up to and during pregnancy. By giving him lots of the right nutrients you give him the perfect building blocks to grow strong and healthy.

Whip up a healthy grilled chicken salad with lots of greens and a few legumes and you're really building a brain and developing a nervous system . . . talk about being a whiz in the kitchen. You don't need to learn how to work blue in the kitchen like Gordon Ramsey or develop a lisp like Jamie Oliver. Simple, fresh and natural foods are all your partner and baby need. We are going to show you which foods do what, so all you need to do is follow some basic guidelines and you'll be growing a baby in no time. It's much more fun than growing a beard or growing old and you'll be able to see the fruits of your labour (pardon the pun) in under nine months!

It's very simple, and it's the best thing you can do to help your baby while he is in the womb. At the end of the chapter we'll provide you with some basic recipes that even a pole-axed monkey (you) could prepare. Imagine your partner's surprise when you dish up a terrific lunch or dinner and give her a lesson in nutrition at the same time.

Nutrition is hardly the stuff you'll find most blokes reading about on the toilet come Sunday morning. We can already sense many of you wanting to skip the next part of this chapter altogether. Even the prospect of building your own baby may not be enough to whet your appetite or keep your eyelids open. So in the interests of your future son or daughter we've listed the 12 essential vitamins and minerals your partner and baby need. Think of them in terms of the best cricket team Australia could field post-war—feel free to email us with reasons why our team should be changed for future editions of this book. We've picked only players and vitamins selected post-war because we never saw the Don wield the willow, and although smoking was considered healthy for the baby when the Jerries were bombing Britain we think we know better now.

The first XII of all-star nutrients you'll need to build your baby

1 Grow me a brain and spinal cord please, Dad— folate or folic acid

Folate is the Matthew Hayden of nutrients: a proven performer who can get your baby's innings off to a solid start. The brain and spinal cord begin life as a neural tube. Now, life without a brain or spinal cord wouldn't be much fun—just ask a plate of raspberry Aeroplane jelly and see what it has to say on the subject.

Your baby needs folate to form its neural tube; without it, there is an increased risk of neural tube defects such as spina bifida. It is recommended that women increase their folate levels in the lead-up to conception and in the first few months of pregnancy. Folate is also required to help with cell division and creation. At around six weeks pregnant the nervous system alone is adding about 100,000 new nerve cells an hour!

You will probably start seeing a pregnancy multivitamin like Elevit appear in your kitchen or bathroom. These multivitamins ensure that she is getting the right amount of the nutrients she needs. If she's not taking a pregnancy multivitamin, discuss it with her.

The best food sources of folate in real food include green beans, leeks, parsnips, cabbage, beetroot, green peas, spinach, capsicum, cauliflower, chickpeas, oranges, orange juice, peanuts, oats and wholegrain bread.

> **TIP**
>
> If it's leafy and green, it's probably got folate on board!

> **FACT**
>
> A woman's folate requirement increases by over 50 per cent during pregnancy.

2   I need muscles and blood—iron, man

There's no good opening the batting with Matthew Hayden and Glenn McGrath. You need a solid opening partner like a Justin Langer. Think of iron as your baby's Justin Langer. Iron and folate are both critical to building your baby's innings.

By month six of the pregnancy your partner has created an extra litre of blood, and by the end she'll be pumping up to 40 per cent more blood than at conception. Your baby also has to create its own blood supply. Iron is the building block for blood. Iron is also required to build muscles and to carry oxygen around the body. Muscles, oxygen and blood . . . yep, he's going to need all of them to play footy.

Good sources of iron include red meat, poultry, fish, cereals, vegetables and legumes (such as dried beans, soybeans, peas and lentils and grains such as oatmeal).

> **FACT**
>
> Vitamin C helps her body to better absorb iron from foods and supplements, so a glass of orange juice a day is a great idea.

3   The brains trust—iodine

We've never worked out why the best cricket captains are generally batsmen and why so many captains bat in the top half of the order. Regardless, iodine is your Alan Border of nutrients: a reliable brains trust who can run the show and still make an impact as an individual.

Iodine will help your baby's thyroid gland function effectively. Hormones produced by the thyroid help with brain, heart, kidney and muscle development. Iodine is important during pregnancy and breastfeeding; iodine deficiency is associated with intellectual impairment.

The best natural sources of iodine are dairy milk, seafood and some table salts that have iodine added. Don't forget to read the 'What she shouldn't eat' section on page 138, though, because some seafood is on the pregnancy equivalent of the anti-doping body's list of banned substances.

4   Sticks and stones may break my bones—because Dad didn't feed me calcium

Unless you've been living in a womb, you probably know that calcium is crucial for strong bones and teeth. We're guessing you don't want to give birth to an invertebrate, so calcium is pretty important. Every team needs a backbone of their innings—a Steve Waugh type of character who can average over 50—and that seems to be calcium.

There is some conjecture as to whether the need for calcium rises in pregnant women or if their body naturally starts absorbing more. Either way it's agreed that it's an essential part of a balanced diet. You can find it in dairy foods (milk, cheese, yoghurt etc.) and cereals.

5   Vitamin B6

This bad boy (think Andrew Symonds) is a real all rounder and responsible for many processes that occur during your baby's development, especially in its nervous system.

Vitamin B6 can be found in bananas, potatoes, watermelon, chickpeas, chicken, red meat and milk.

FACT and TIP

An increase in vitamin B6 has been shown to help minimise morning sickness in some women.

---

6   Zinc

Zinc is another all rounder of the mineral world. Let's think of it as the Adam Gilchrist in our squad of essential nutrients.

Zinc can be found in just about every cell of your baby's body. It helps your baby develop a healthy immune system and a sense of smell and taste . . . not that he probably wants one while swallowing amniotic fluid in his nine-month stay in the womb! A lack of zinc may lead to premature birth and slowed growth. No thanks.

Good sources of zinc include beef, lamb, pork, crabmeat, turkey, chicken, lobster, salmon, milk and cheese, yeast, peanuts, beans, wholegrain cereals, brown rice, whole wheat bread, potato and yoghurt.

7 Chromium—not of the bumper bar variety

The number 7 position is often a difficult position for the selectors to fill. All rounder, specialist bowler or extra batsman? With Gilly in the team and a world-class bowling line-up we could probably not even have a number 7 and still beat any team going around. For good measure we'll throw Boony in (yes, we know he was a number three batsman), because chromium can be found in beer and with Boony around there will always be a solid beer supply on hand. Not that we condone alcoholic beverages for pregnant women but you'll need to make sure your chromium levels stay up there as well . . . hem, hem!

Chromium is necessary for regulating your partner's blood sugar levels and it stimulates the synthesis of protein in your growing baby's tissues. You can find it in peanut butter, spinach, mushrooms and wholegrain bread, but we wouldn't suggest all those ingredients in a wholegrain bread sandwich. You can probably also go to the summer nats in Canberra and make your partner lick a lot of bumper bars if you're a cheapskate.

8 Omega 3 fatty acids—Warney?

Warney is infamous for his Hawaiian pizza, baked beans and Escort Blue diet, none of which contains any omega 3 fatty acids. These essential building blocks are critical for brain development—a function sometimes called into question with Shane. In adults they help keep your heart and immune system healthy. All in all they are an indispensable part of the nutrient line-up—much like the great spinner himself.

Shane, for the record, omega 3 fatty acids can be found in oily fish such as mackerel and salmon, flax seeds, walnuts, vegetable oils (such as canola oil or soybean oil) and to a lesser extent in eggs and meat.

> ## FACT
>
> Your brain is 60 per cent fat. Now you know why you've been told you have a fat head.

9, 10, 11 and 12   Niacin, riboflavin, thiamine and pantothenic acid

Where would you be without a quality bowling attack? As with your opening batsmen you need a cohesive unit, a trio of quicks who share the workload and get through the vital task at hand. Glenn McGrath, Dennis Lilley and Jason Gillespie come to mind, with Merv Hughes carrying the drinks just in case.

Most of these minerals sound poisonous to us and hardly five-star dining fare, but they are required. They work in unison and are 'co-enzymes active in a variety of metabolic processes'. Let's just leave it at that.

Niacin can be found in whole grains, legumes, nuts, meat, fish and poultry. Riboflavin bobs up in whole grains, milk, meats and liver and thiamine resides in whole grains and pork. Pantothenic acid is in whole grains, yeast, potatoes, tomatoes, eggs, broccoli, chicken and beef.

*   *   *

Now you know what are the basic building blocks required to build your baby and impress your partner. However, like a Lego set without instructions, the information is probably completely useless to you. Stay tuned and we'll introduce you to Lisa Neal who will provide you with a few recipes to help you out.

Don't forget that good food isn't important just for your baby. Your partner is going through enormous physical changes and certain foods can help her with common pregnancy ailments like fatigue, nausea, constipation, cramps, indigestion . . . and a deep-rooted hatred of you!

Pregnancy supplements

Many nutrients play somewhat similar roles and scientists and other boffins are discovering new stuff every day about what role certain nutrients play in baby development.

Pregnancy supplements/multivitamins are a great insurance policy for your baby but they are not a substitute for a nutrient-rich diet. Most pregnancy supplements contain all the goodies listed above and more, including vitamins B, C and E, magnesium and others. Your partner should speak with her medical practitioner or dietician about a suitable multivitamin for her.

It's also worth remembering that the amount of nutrients in supplements isn't always of the same value as what you would get from real food. For example, 1 gram of folate in a pregnancy supplement is only worth about 500 milligrams (that is, half) of folate consumed through real food.

Eating right isn't an option, it's a necessity. Build your baby using the best possible fuel at all times.

What she shouldn't eat

We're certain that most women worry more about what they shouldn't eat than about what they should. Yes, some foods are considered not ideal for the baby, but if you listened to what everyone had to say you'd be living on a diet of glacial water flown in from the Antarctic in penguin bladders and the livers of mountain goats from the Chilean town of Los Stupidos.

Testing positive for the following items will get your partner sent home from the pregnancy world cup, Shane Warne style. You don't want her blaming you for giving these to her . . . you will be despised by the nation.

1 Cigarettes

Imagine being down at the local Westfield shopping centre, sipping on your decaf soy frappacino and seeing a mum stick a lit cigarette in a newborn's mouth. Now imagine that same baby smoking it, sucking all that crap into its tiny lungs and flicking the cigarette butt onto the ground and butting it out with his home-knitted woollen booty. Shocking. Well, that's exactly what is happening if your partner smokes during pregnancy.

But we're not smokers and have no experience at going cold turkey on them. Clearly it's no picnic, so if your partner is/was a smoker and you are too, do everyone a favour and quit when she does.

2 Booze

There are two schools of thought on this one:

1. complete abstinence; and
2. an occasional glass of wine is OK.

There is no doubt that serious alcohol intake harms a baby. You only need to see an image of a baby with foetal alcohol syndrome to swear off the VB for life. Speak to your doctor and discuss your position on it with your partner.

Just because she's pregnant doesn't mean she won't be longing for a beverage. Comb the community forums of any big pregnancy website and you will see women discussing how they are longing for a cocktail and how much they despise us for getting on the beer at every opportunity because we have a designated driver.

If you were the best bloke in the world you'd give up drinking during her pregnancy, but chances are that you're not the best bloke in the world and won't give up drinking, so at least try to be sympathetic on this one.

3   Caffeine

The fun police seem to believe coffee should also be on the banned list, but other sources say the occasional cup is OK. One dad we met remembers being eighteen and stepping off an overnight train from Paris to Florence and ordering an Italian espresso. It was his first ever coffee and despite the fact that it was served in a thimble, its effect was not unlike that of amphetamines . . . it sent him straight to the toilet and then the dance floor. If even a small amount of caffeine crosses through the placenta to the baby we can't help thinking it would have a similar effect. We're not card-carrying members of the fun police, though, so you make up your own mind.

4   Mercury–loving fish

Fish naturally accumulate mercury, and some species do so more than others. Fish are a great source of protein, minerals, vitamin B12 and iodine and are low in saturated fat, so including them in your diet is recommended. Stick to mackerel, salmon, whiting and garfish and eat no more than two or three serves a week. They are four of the tastiest fish in the ocean, so why go elsewhere! If she doesn't like fish, look for a good Omega 3 supplement (one that uses mercury-free fish).

5   Soft cheese and uncooked meats

These bad boys can harbour listeria, which sounds more like a mouth freshener than a baby killer. So it's no brie and prosciutto toasted sandwiches for the next nine months. And if you're preparing meat and fish, make sure you give it an extra few minutes on the BBQ and cook it through.

Eating for 1.2

By now you'll be familiar with old pregnancy chestnuts like 'Don't do that, you're just making a rod for your own back' and 'No wonder she's hungry, she's eating for two now!' We still don't know what making a rod for your own back is or why anyone, other than invertebrates, would do it, but we have learned that eating for two is complete bollocks. In reality your partner is eating for 1.2 at the most and she only needs an extra 300 or so calories a day, which is bugger all.

What she does have a need for is an increase in nutrients so the extra 300 calories need to be nutrient rich, not a Mars bar. Now is the time to take stock of what you're both eating and what you're going to eat for the next eight months. Organic food is the way to go but it can be difficult to find in many places and can also be quite expensive. Try to eat fresh produce, and think about how to get as many natural nutrients into mum and baby as possible. The Shane Warne diet is certainly not recommended by the surgeon general.

We'll cover cravings and weight gain in the next chapter.

Who ate all the pies?

If you're like most guys, you're quite likely to 'go out in sympathy' in the weight department. In the next chapter we will have a look at Couvade syndrome (page 166), which is the phenomenon of men experiencing pregnancy symptoms when their partner is pregnant. The reality is that in the coming months you're at serious risk of entering a kilo addition program. Why? Here are a few possible reasons:

- Her appetite may wane and you might eat your pork chops and hers for a few months . . . and her Sara Lee apple turnover with double lashings of cream.

- She may have cravings for sugary or fatty foods . . . why should you deny yourself the late night pleasure of a deep-fried Mars bar?

- She's tired and not feeling like exercise . . . it's a great excuse to stay on the couch and watch the footy.

- She's massive and can't see her feet let alone fit through the turnstile at the gym . . . see point three.
- She's driving you nuts and to drink . . . better stock up on the low-carb beers.

The first few months of parenthood can be bedlam, and chances are you won't feel like working out. Eating well and exercise are vital in keeping fit and healthy and in helping you survive less sleep and more stress. Getting yourselves into good shape now and maintaining that through early parenthood will deliver many benefits.

Cooking—it's not a dirty word and it's way sexier than vacuuming

Long gone are the days when the kitchen is the domain of women. If you've not been one for donning the apron and wielding the steel in the kitchen, now is a great time to learn. Cooking is considered a domestic chore but it's a lot more enjoyable than ironing, picking up dirty clothes or vacuuming (unless you have a ride-on vacuum cleaner). Plus, you can have a beer while cooking and watch sport on TV while cooking, and it's impressive to all members of the female race (much more so than ironing pillowcases).

As we discussed in Chapter 2, you're going to have to start upping the ante on the domestic chore front. We put it to you that cooking is the single most fun chore one can do inside the house. It's also a fabulous skill to have once the kids are older and can cook with you, and for when your partner leaves you (so you don't starve to death or get as fat as a house from eating takeaway food every night).

If you really want to get extra brownie points before the baby comes, sign yourself and your partner up for a few cooking classes. They can be great fun and a genuinely good date night out. Oh, and most courses serve beer or wine during and after . . . that's a bonus.

Baby making recipes with Lisa Neal

To make it easy for you to whip together a few simple dishes we've enlisted the help of Lisa Neal, author of the fabulous book *Feeding the Bump*. Lisa isn't a chef or a dietitian but wanted to help dads-to-be get into the kitchen and start building babies. Her book is a new dad's best friend and has great recipes for different stages of the pregnancy. It is the perfect guide to building a baby for every dad-to-be.

We were looking at creating a *Being Dad* cookbook but Lisa beat us to the punch and her book is so good we decided we couldn't top it. Grab yourself a copy.

Lisa kindly lent us a few recipes, though, so blokes—get cooking!

Seafood Stew

This is probably one of the easiest, tastiest and nourishing recipes you could cook for your partner. It provides close to all of the nutrients essential to a healthy pregnancy and is particularly rich in zinc and iodine. It is very easy to become deficient in these two nutrients, and yet they are vital to normal and proper development of the brain and central nervous system. The stew is also rich in omega 3 and protein. Put simply, this dish is brain food for your partner and baby.

1 leek or large brown onion
3 garlic cloves, crushed
1 tbs olive oil
½ tsp sweet paprika
1 × 400 g canned diced tomatoes
½ cup water
2 bay leaves
2 tsp dried thyme
black pepper

10 fresh mussels, in their shells
1 snapper fillet
1 salmon fillet
100 g calamari rings
½ cup fresh parsley, finely chopped

Finely slice the leek/onion and prepare the garlic.

Heat the olive oil in a heavy-based frying pan with a lid. Cook the leeks/onion for 4–5 minutes, or until soft. Add the garlic and cook for a further 2 minutes before adding the paprika and continue cooking for another minute or two. Add the tomatoes, water, bay leaves and thyme. Season generously with black pepper. Bring the sauce to a gentle simmer, cover and cook for 10 minutes.

Meanwhile, prepare the seafood. Place the mussels in a colander and rinse under cold running water. Thoroughly scrub the mussel shells to remove any barnacles and pull out the 'hairy beards'. Discard any mussels with cracked shells. Give them a final rinse with cold water and leave to drain.

Cut the fish fillets into 3-centimetre pieces, removing the skin and any bones. Combine with the calamari rings.

Once the tomato mixture has cooked for 10 minutes, add the seafood. Gently stir through and coat with the sauce. Cover the pan and cook for 5–7 minutes, shaking the pan once or twice.

Check to see if the fish is cooked through. Remove the bay leaves and any mussels that have not opened. Dislodge the mussels from their shells. Discard the shells and add the mussels to the stew.

Stir through fresh parsley and serve with a small bowl of steamed greens and crusty wholegrain bread to soak up the seafood broth.

Barbecue Lamb Fillets with Mushy Peas

This is a perfect example of eating the nutrients for two and it is not a stretch to say that this is a completely balanced meal. You might be surprised to learn that lamb contains more iron than beef. And the pea belongs to the legume family and is incredibly nutrient rich; it contains eight vitamins, plus minerals and loads of dietary fibre. Peas also have a low GI rating to help maintain blood sugar levels and reduce the risk of developing many of the common complaints of pregnancy.

400 g lean lamb backfillets
olive oil for basting
lots of cracked black pepper
400 g frozen peas
2 tbs fresh mint
2 tbs low fat plain yoghurt
2 tsp olive oil

Preheat a barbecue or grill to a medium heat. Trim the lamb of any excess fat and lightly baste with the olive oil and season with the pepper. Place the lamb on the barbecue or grill and cook for 4 minutes on each side or until cooked through. Set aside in a warm place and let the lamb rest for a couple of minutes before serving.

While the lamb is cooking, add the peas to boiling water and cook for 3–4 minutes. Drain and put the peas into a food processor together with the mint and yoghurt. Process for a minute or two, scrape the peas from the side, add the olive oil and process for a further minute or so until you have a puree consistency. I like to have a few chunky peas in mine, but you might like yours smooth. Season generously with black pepper.

Place a large dollop of the peas in the centre of each plate and top with the lamb fillets.

For a heartier meal, serve with baked sweet potato chips. Simply cut sweet potato into thick cubes, place on a sheet of baking paper and cook in a pre-heated oven for 40 minutes.

Berry Blast

This is great for preconception, first trimester and breastfeeding. Enjoy for breakfast, between meals or even as a dessert. It is rich in anti-oxidants to boost the immune system and prime the mother's body for the nine months ahead and is a great meal option when nauseous and solids are hard to tolerate.

1 banana
½ cup frozen blueberries
3–4 ice cubes
1/3 cup (80 ml) skim/soy milk
1 tbs skim milk powder
½ cup plain yoghurt/soy yoghurt
1 tbs wheatgerm

Place the fruit and ice into a blender and process for 30 seconds.

Add the remaining ingredients, blend until smooth and serve immediately.

(Recipes courtesy of *Feeding the Bump*)

Exercising—preparing your partner and baby for the marathon of birth

Now it's time to start helping your partner prepare for the marathon of childbirth. Birth has been likened to taking a very brisk 6-kilometre walk in terms of the energy that is used in the process. That's fairly staggering when you consider how little distance she'll actually be covering and that she'll already be exhausted, emotional and almost literally bursting at the seams!

Exercise plays a huge role in the health of mum and baby during pregnancy and prepares them both for the rigours of birth. You wouldn't go out and run a marathon without some serious preparation, so why would you go into a similarly demanding and important event like childbirth underdone?

How exercise helps build your baby and prepare your partner for birth

In centuries gone by we were all a lot more active by necessity. Sitting behind a computer screen and shopping at Woolworths weren't options, so we had to work hard physically. That much more active lifestyle was very good for physically preparing women's bodies for childbirth.

In their book *The Natural Way to Better Birthing and Bonding*, Nash and Roberts list the benefits of exercise:

- Better delivery of nutrients and oxygen to the placenta and baby—getting your food to him!
- More efficient circulation and better blood pressure for mum.
- Less likelihood of varicose veins—yes, please.
- Improved stamina and endurance.
- A shorter and easier labour—we'll take two of those!
- Easing of pain during labour and easier passage for the baby.
- Decreased risk of tearing.
- Faster recovery after birth.

To us this means it helps build your baby and makes birth easier and more enjoyable, so pass us the Nikes!

Exercise can throw up a few emotional issues as well:

- If your partner is an exercise nut and has to wind back her regime, she may become stressed by not being able to work out with her normal fervour and she may want to get back into exercising too soon after birth.

- If your partner has high blood pressure or other health problems and is unable to exercise, she may start getting stressed at having to be sedentary.
- If your partner has never exercised and is pressured into it, she may feel resentful.

You know your partner, so if you think one of the above may apply talk with her about it and talk to your doctor about how best to handle your situation.

What exercises can she do and what can you help with?

Cardiovascular/aerobic workouts

These are designed to get the ticker working and the blood pumping, and all you need to do is go for brisk walks together.

Starting an exercise regime early in the pregnancy allows you to get into a routine together. Aim for three or four 30–40 minute walks per week. Check with your doctor first that exercising is OK. As the pregnancy progresses, the extra weight puts a load on joints and muscles so it's important to not overdo any exercise.

Muscle strengthening

Building up her muscles will help her cope with carrying the baby around. Try on an empathy belly, which simulates carrying a near-term baby, and you will soon feel how the extra weight puts strain on your legs, arse, abdomen and back. Unless you're a qualified instructor it's probably best to sign her up for a gym or pregnancy fitness class.

Muscle conditioning helps during pregnancy and with birth.

Pelvic floor exercises

Have you ever heard of Dr Arnold Kegel? Us neither. Turns out old Arnie was a gynaecologist who invented a device that could measure vaginal air pressure and exercises to strengthen the muscles of the pelvic floor—these exercises are now known as Kegel exercises.

Vaginal air pressure . . . we think Rolex could use that on their next women's aviator wristwatch. Just imagine the benefits of knowing the time and the PSI in your private bits . . . hard to imagine why it hasn't taken off sooner.

Back to the pelvic floor. For men, exercising pelvic floor muscles can help reduce urinary incontinence and prostate pain and increase sexual gratification (stronger erections and the ability to delay orgasms for longer). Clearly, you should know something about the big K, and maybe even practise along with your partner!

If you've ever been having sex and had the girl 'grip' you from the inside, she's probably familiar with Dr Kegel. Old Doc Kegel also came up with a Kegel exerciser which looks like a modified metal dildo . . . maybe he knew what he was up to after all.

Pelvic floor muscles are used during childbirth and, like any muscles, exercising makes them stronger and more resilient. By strengthening her pelvic floor muscles your partner can also reduce the risk of tearing during birth.

Your childbirth class should provide instruction on Kegel exercises, which is a good reason to attend.

WARNING WARNING DEFCON 4 ALERT

If you're thinking the Kegel exercises are too good to be true, you're right. Any recommendations to get on board with Kegel exercises are likely to be accompanied with advice on perineum stretching. The perineum is the bit between the vagina and the bum and perineum stretching is advisable in the weeks leading up to the birth to help prevent tearing.

You may be asked to participate in the perineum stretching process. It will be very helpful for her, but may also be very stressful for you! The prospect of stretching your partner's vagina isn't something most men will leap at, so maybe while she's doing her stretching you can be in the kitchen making one of Lisa's recipes from *Feeding the Bump*.

Practising birth positions

In Chapter 8 we look at birthing positions that your partner can use to help give her and the baby an easier birth. You, our friend, will help her with these positions. You will need to know them, and to encourage her to try different positions as labour progresses.

These positions include squatting, kneeling and standing, and all of them require good muscle strength to pull them off. So practising these positions during pregnancy is not only doing a trial run for the big day, but also helping her strengthen the right muscles. Don't forget, she'll be a lot heavier then, so the muscles will need time to adjust to her increasing weight.

If all of this sounds ridiculous and a waste of time, just ask yourself this: Do you want your birth to be as enjoyable, painless (for Mum, baby and you) and as memorable as possible? If the answer is yes, start exercising today—tomorrow if you're reading this in bed.

*   *   *

Helping your partner eat well and exercise are the two biggest ways that you can directly influence the health and development of your baby. It's your first role as being a dad.

Congratulations, you are now qualified to build your baby.

It's not an official qualification so don't add it to your curriculum vitae, but you now know the only physical way that you can have a positive effect on the development, growth and health of your baby. We don't have any empirical proof to back this up, but we believe that if you understand the benefits of nutrition and exercise and you cook for her (and the baby) and exercise with her it will help you start to form a bond with your baby.

Later we will discuss other ways to bond with your baby in utero. In the meantime, head to the kitchen, grab a beer and get cooking!

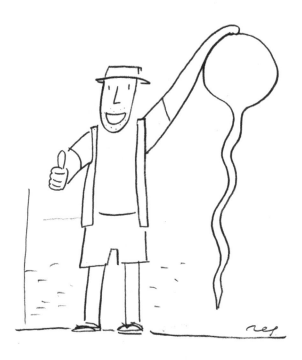

Chapter 7

Trimester 3

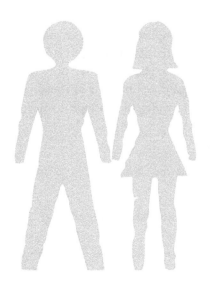

FOR H✝R

By now your man should be starting to shape up as a concerned, helpful, understanding, committed partner and dad-to-be. Up until now he's had it pretty easy: we've been opening the door ever so slightly and shining a thin beam of light into that once nebulous void. The realities of what lie ahead have shifted from the DENIAL file across to the PENDING file. Sure, it's a slow process, but the internal wiring of your man, as you've come to learn, is complicated: snip the blue wire instead of the red wire and BOOM, you're back to square one.

From here on we will turn the thumb screws a little tighter, push the door ajar and turn the lights on—it's time for him to step up. Parenting classes, babyproofing the house, nursery shopping, birth plan creation, hospital visits, hot dates and, dare we say it, perineum stretching are all on the cards. We only have 90 days, or 2160 hours, until the due date and half of those will be spent sleeping (or trying to get comfortable enough to sleep). The pressure is on.

What's on his mind in T3?

Paternity

Is the baby his? Well, only you know the answer to that. No matter how much your partner trusts you, there is likely to be some point during or after the pregnancy when the question will cross his mind. We're not certain if it's a defensive mechanism, his inner wild beast talking or just his wild imagination, but it's a reality for many first-time dads.

In a few surveys we've read, the answer to 'Did you ever think the baby wasn't yours?' was 'Yes' for as high as 65 per cent, but when we conducted our own poll among Aussie dads the figure was 18 per cent. You know if this is a subject worth broaching with your man; the point is, don't be totally shocked if at some point the subject arises.

The health of you and the baby

We seem to be a very nervous breed these days, and pregnancy and birth have become more a medical complication than a natural process. The internet, TV and other media expose us all too often to what can go wrong during childbirth and pregnancy. In 2010 the new buzz is about kick counts, and we saw our first kick counter on the weekend. It's a tiny device you hold on your belly and it counts how many times junior bear sinks in the boot. We can already see the issues a device like this will raise in those of a nervous disposition.

Your man will start worrying about your health and the baby's, but probably he will be focused more on the actual birth. Men are born with an 'I'm sure it's fine, let's wait until the morning' attitude and you can expect to hear this whenever you complain during T3. It's not that he is insensitive; he is just trying to keep you relaxed and calm.

You know your body, and if you feel something isn't right of course you should call your doctor—we will do our best to drum that into him!

Coping with the birth

If it's his first child or he's had a previous bad experience he will probably be concerned, even scared, about his ability to cope with the birth. As we've already discussed, watching you in pain and witnessing the anatomical side of birth isn't easy for the faint of heart!

It's important to create a birth plan together and to discuss what you'd like him to do with you during the birth and what he is comfortable doing.

It's our experience that most guys are surprised at their ability to cope when the time comes. Somehow, once you're in the heat of battle it does become a natural process, and the male mind manages to do what it does best: switch off. We will arm him with instructions on how he can make the experience better for you both—we advise developing a birth plan after he has read this chapter.

You and the nest

At the risk of generalising, it's probably fair to suggest that most first-time pregnant women get a little giddy at the prospect of buying kiddies' stuff, and that's even before the nesting instincts kick into overdrive. The maternity market is huge and they are exceptionally good at bombarding you with crap you don't need. The temptation is to fill your cupboards with cute clothes, buy strollers that are worth more than most small cars and collect an endless array of totally useless bits and pieces, most of which are plastic and have a half-life of plutonium.

We implore you to set a budget, shop wisely and involve him in at least some of the decision making. To honour the code of blokesmanship we have given him a list of essentials and of things that you don't need. We know you'll hate us for it but come on—we've been on your side the whole way so far. Forgive us this one indulgence!

Getting him to childbirth classes

We're sorry, but those two words strike fear into the heart of every man. We've been conditioned by those who leapt over the trenches before us that they are boring, time-consuming, irrelevant and a pain in the arse. Fortunately for you, the good folks at *Being Dad* set about righting that ship a while back and sent free copies of our DVDs to every childbirthing class in the country in the hope that they would start also focusing on dads.

We've had great feedback and we know there are lots of educators who now also include dads into the classes and play clips from our DVDs, so the word is spreading slowly that they aren't so bad after all. Nevertheless, here are some tips to help you lock and load your man for the childbirth experience:

- Book the classes early and put the dates in every calendar he ever looks at.
- Remind him weekly/monthly when the classes are.
- Look into classes with him, ask him what he wants to know and what he'd prefer timewise (weekends or weeknights).

In these last few months it's important to continue to work on your relationship to make sure your expectations, goals and hopes are aligned. Keep reassuring him that things will be OK and that he'll be a good dad. Spend some time with friends who have small kids and try to have his male friends talk to him about the realities of fatherhood. Make time to spend together and if possible have a few weekend getaways.

Now it's time to hand the book over to him.

FOR HIM

Righto chaps, if this were military recruit training you'd have had your head shaved, been issued your khakis and been given a lesson in how to really swear by now.

SAM: My brief time in the army did provide me with some insight into pregnancy and birth. It's tough to erase the memory of my drill sergeant screaming in my face on a 40 degrees Celcius day in Wagga Wagga, 'Recruit Holt, if you f+ck up once more I'll poke your eye out, skull fuck you and you can be the father of my brainchild.' Fortunately I made it off the drill square with both eyes and my skull's virginity intact . . . but I've never recovered mentally.

It's time to get down to business, learn what life's really like in the trenches, how to dress a sucking chest wound in the field and drink your own urine when the water supply lines have been cut.

It's two trimesters down and only one to go. Time is running out and there is much to do and cram in. It's not all bad news; in this chapter we are going to save you thousands of dollars in unnecessary purchases and teach you how to be battle ready for the birth. By the time you hit the birth chapter you'll be ready to stare fatherhood, and your new nipper, in the eye.

Her retail therapy—nesting isn't only for birds

We have a horrible habit of calling women birds, and they really hate it. That has nothing to do with this topic other than to say your bird will probably experience the need to nest in T3. Nesting can take on many forms, from insisting that a set square and spirit level be used when setting up the nursery to cleaning anything and everything and looking to spend the GDP of a small African nation on useless crap none of you need.

On the cleaning and nursery front we suggest you let her run wild, but when it comes to the purchasing of baby items we suggest you get involved.

Becoming a parent for the first time can become a very expensive experience. Many couples want to have everything new for the first baby, so there is a tendency to go overboard and spend way more than you need to. The baby industry is a behemoth and has become very savvy at targeting new mums. In the baby world, branding is everywhere and marketers use celebrity endorsements to make certain items seem essential. Take your humble stroller. When we were kids, strollers were pretty basic fold-up items that were used solely as a back-saving device. These days, strollers are fashion accessories and come with more features than the latest BMW 3 series and a price tag to match.

The stroller is just one of the thousands of items that your partner will be told she must have. Almost none of these essentials existed when we were babies, and while some are valuable additions many are a complete waste of time, money and space.

Following is a list of kit that should go on the YES list, a heap of crap for the NO list and some other bits and pieces you can forage from friends and family. You may have hit the roof when your partner paid yet more cold, hard cash for this book, but it's about to save you hundreds if not thousands of dollars.

Stuff you do not need

- *A nappy bag that has bunnies on it.* Nappy bags are pretty handy, but get something you can both use and something that you can use after the baby. You'll be surprised just how handy these things are when you find yourself covered in vomit or poo in the park, and how impressed other mums are when you whip open your kit bag and clean up the mess, then feed and change the baby, then retrieve your smoked salmon bagel and thermos of piping hot coffee, all with effortless ease.
- *A big, expensive stroller.* There's a good chance she'll want the Rolls Royce Silver Shadow of strollers. Make sure you get involved in the purchasing decision so you can apply your man logic to it. If you're into your exercise you definitely want to get involved, because getting the right model is imperative for running and easy pushing. The truth is that in the early months it's great to carry your baby in a sling or papoose. Save the stroller decision for later, once you have a better idea of your parenting style.

- *Small receiving blankets.* The extra large ones work better for swaddling, burps and keeping baby covered (and they can be used for years because your child won't grow too big for them for a long while).
- *Too many pieces of baby clothing.* You don't know what size your baby will be when it's born and you may not know the gender. Nippers grow so bloody fast they are in and out of new clothes in the blink of an eye. You can easily drop $100 on a baby outfit that gets worn once . . . or not even once.
- *Plastic baby bottles, cups, plates, bowls and spoons that have bisphenol-A, phthalates or lead in them.* You'll get given plenty of baby stuff, so just concentrate on what you'll need for the first month or two and then see what comes your way.

Stuff worth having

- *A new baby seat for the car.* This is not an area to scrimp and save on. Get a car seat that is easy to install and use and comes with the best safety rating available. It pays to have said car seat professionally installed (well in advance!). You'll never live it down if you're racing off to the emergency ward without a fitted car seat!
- *A sling or baby carrier.* You can wear your baby. Babies cry less when close to you, so go hands-free and you'll both be happier. A man with a new baby in a sling or baby carrier is the greatest chick magnet on earth (except maybe that same bloke with a Labrador puppy). Not that you need or want to be a chick magnet these days, but it's still nice to know you've got it.
- *A healthier crib mattress.* Flame retardants and the plastics used in some mattresses and other baby items give off fumes that are not good for you or your baby's health. Try a wool-covered or latex mattress.
- *Breast pumps.* If you do get a breast pump, go electric and choose a pump made by a company that specialises in them.

When it comes to expressing, you will both want it to be just that: 'express'. The last thing you want in the middle of the night is for the baby to be sleeping soundly but the two of you lying awake as she manually pumps breast milk.

- *Toys that are made from healthier plastics, wood and cloth (batteries not needed!).* Put a ban on plastic toys from friends and family. The last thing you need is a house cluttered with plastic toys that will barely get used and take up a load of space.

- *A good quality ear thermometer.* Little kids seem to always be running a temperature, and you'll want to know when they are just hot as opposed to when they are boiling over. Being a first-time parent can be really frightening when your little one gets sick. A good baby first aid class is really worthwhile. Many good birthing classes should also give you some education on this front.

- *A cupboard full of baby Panadol!* It should go without saying that you must check with your doctor before giving your baby any medication, but when they are running a temperature this stuff is like liquid gold. It really pays to have it accessible at all times and in all places.

Stuff worth getting from friends and family

Whatever you can! Just make sure that it's in a good state of repair and clean.

Childbirth classes

These two words will strike fear into the heart of any self-respecting bloke. The consensus among new dads is that you do, unfortunately, have to attend. Below are some questions that will help you choose a class that won't make you want to top yourself.

1. *Do I have to go?* This is NOT a question to ask . . . unless you like the bite of a seething, hormonally charged, pregnant viper.

2. *How many couples will be in the class (maximum)?* We recommend a class with nine or fewer couples. It makes it more interactive and you're more likely to get your questions heard and answered.

3. *Are there handouts?* Most adults are better learners if they see it, hear it and do it. Use them to your advantage—your partner needs your help remembering everything (remember baby brain?).

4. *What kind of activities will we do in class?* Look for a class that gets you moving and practising techniques for labour.

5. *Do they involve dads in their classes?* You're BOTH having a baby, so you shouldn't feel you're just along for the ride. You're super important in this process!

6. *What other classes are offered?* Newborn care, breastfeeding, CPR and others are also important classes to take so you both feel ready for the new and most important job you've ever had. You wouldn't start a new job in a new career without some training, would you?

7. *How long do classes run?* One-day classes can't give you all the info and practice you'll need to be truly prepared for birth; natural childbirth classes should be even longer. These longer classes give you a chance to really practise relaxation techniques, positions, massage, using tools for labour (like nubby dog toys, tennis balls and Play-doh!).

Ask your buddies. Find one or two who really loved their class and consider taking classes with those childbirth educators!

BELIEVE US: when you find yourself in the midst of active labour and the delivery, you'll be glad you went to the classes.

A few things you MUST do this trimester

Having surveyed hundreds of new dads around the world, here is a list of tasks that we think every dad MUST complete between now and the birth. As you have no idea whether the baby may come early, it pays to get stuck in and do these as early as possible:

1   Choose and install a car seat for the baby and have it inspected by a certified child passenger safety technician (car seat inspector)

Choosing a car seat can be mind-boggling. Do your research and make sure you're comfortable with the one you've chosen. Have a look on www.choice.com.au.

If you plan to get a used car seat from a friend or relative, only get it from someone you trust entirely. Ask them if the car has been in a car accident with the car seat in it. If it has, don't use the seat. Check the date on the bottom of the seat to make sure it's not expired. Also check that it has an Australian Standard number, and that the standard is still current.

Having the seat installed is your domain. Have it installed and inspected in advance (some hospitals have an installing service; if not, they'll tell you where to find one). This is serious stuff. Some hospitals will not let you take the baby home if the car seat isn't properly installed.

2   Help set up the crib and paint the nursery

Your partner is in nesting mode (or will be soon), and nothing will make her feel more prepared than seeing the baby's room set up in advance. If you're like most guys you'll want to leave it until the last minute, but when the baby comes you'll want to be at the hospital, not at home stuffing up the crib. Don't forget to get baby-friendly paint!!

3   *Organise a few hot dates*

This will be the last chance to spend time as just the two of you for a long time. Surprise her by taking her out on a date somewhere special. And a pregnancy massage is a good idea!

4   *Consider a 'push present' (that is, a present before the birth)*

In some countries it is becoming common for men to give their partners a 'push present'. It could be something small, like cooking a nice dinner, arranging a schedule for people to come and help her after the baby's arrival or even a nice piece of jewellery. Mums love gifts, especially gifts that show you appreciate what she endured to help create your new family. A present isn't necessary, of course, but it's sure to win you maximum brownie points, and you'll probably need them soon!

5   *Childproof your house—for your baby's safety and your sanity*

Your baby won't be crawling around for several months, but it's a great idea to get the safety items in place now. Children under the age of four have the highest rate of accidental death among children. It pays to safeguard your house before birth. See our tips for childproofing your home on page 165.

6   *Get your butt into a child education class*

7   *Write down a list of all important numbers (doctors, midwives, the hospital etc.)*

Make sure you have them in your mobile phone and stuck on the fridge; if an emergency arises you'll be wanting those numbers pronto.

8   *Get some time in with your mates*

Eleven tips for childproofing your home

1. Ensure all rubbish containers have lids that can be securely fastened.

2. Install child locks on drawers and cupboards in the kitchen, bathroom and laundry.

3. Keep chemicals and cleaning agents out of reach (even better, switch to all-natural non-toxic cleaning products such as vinegar and baking soda).

4. Install safety bars and locks on the windows in your baby's room.

5. Ensure that smoke detectors are installed and operational.

6. Lower the hot water temperature to 49°C.

7. Install screens around electric, bar and gas heaters.

8. Get non-slip mats for the kitchen and bathroom floors.

9. Install child-resistant outlet plugs.

10. Make sure your TV is firmly anchored and shelves can't be pulled down by a little one.

11. Prepare any pets for the arrival of a new flatmate (see Chapter 12).

Six warning signs during pregnancy and early labour

When it comes to pregnancy, women have pretty good intuition about their body and what is happening to it.

Living in Australia, we have an abundance of really great health care available—if you live in a city or major town, it's likely to be not very far from your front door. If either of you is doubtful about something, check it out. Forget your blokey tendencies: not wanting to bother people, thinking that you will be a nuisance. The medical staff are there to help, and you're better off asking for directions sooner rather than later. People will take you seriously and are very happy to help.

You'll soon find out, if you don't already know it, that your partner has a much higher tolerance to pain than you do, so if she starts complaining or experiences the following in the later stages of pregnancy or during early labour, call her medical caregiver immediately:

1. A fever above 37°C.

2. Downstairs bleeding.

3. A sense that the baby isn't moving the way it usually does at a particular time of day or night.

4. Just not feeling right (don't try to convince her she's fine; she might be, but it's better to suggest that she talk to her medical caregiver).

5. Vomiting and/or diarrhoea that doesn't go away (and an inability to keep liquids down).

6. A burning sensation when she pees.

There is a phenomenon known as Couvade syndrome that occurs with some men during pregnancy; it's when men experience pregnancy symptoms, from morning sickness right through to labour pains!! There has been quite a bit of research done into whether Couvade syndrome is real or just men's way of seeking attention. Based on what we've read we're tipping the latter—it's a bit like that old chestnut of dogs looking like their owners and vice versa. If you start experiencing early labour pains it's probably time to toughen up. You most certainly are not about to go into labour, and unless your appendix is about to implode you're not in any medical danger.

Signs of premature labour

Premature labour is one of the scariest possibilities for a first-time dad and mum. Unfortunately, lads, it does happen, because it really is the baby who decides when to come out and meet you guys.

Everyone has seen pictures of a tiny premature baby with tubes up its nose. The reality is that modern medical techniques have vastly improved the way we look after premature babies. Babies have been born as early as 22–24 weeks and been completely fine once they leave the neonatal ward.

It is a serious situation, but the nurses, doctors and midwives of the country are experienced professionals and have dealt with it before. Get to your hospital quickly and safely, but try to stay as calm as possible. It truly is miraculous how much can be done to help premature babies become just as healthy as the on-timers.

A premature birth can mean that you and your partner will not get to take your baby home for a while. Having to say goodnight and then sleep away from your baby each night will take a toll on you both.

Thirteen steps to take in the very rare case of an emergency birth

If your partner goes into labour and everything happens so quickly that you have to deliver the baby, here's what you need to do:

1. STAY CALM and stay with your partner. She will very likely be frightened too. The more relaxed and reassured everyone is, the better the result. Fake the coolness if you have to.

2. If you were planning on birthing in a hospital or birth centre, call 000 and they will send emergency medical technicians; if you were planning a home birth, call your midwife.

3. Where possible, wash your hands thoroughly and gather clean towels and bed sheets.

4. Reassure your partner that you're there for her and that everything will be OK.

5. Help your partner find a comfortable birth position (on her knees bending forward, squatting or lying on her side are the most comfortable positions for most women).

6. Look for the baby's head.

7. When the head is visible, ask your partner to stop pushing and just blow.

8. After the baby's head is out, feel around the baby's neck to ensure that the umbilical cord is not wrapped around it. If it is, stay calm and hook your fingers under the cord and gently loop it around the baby's head.

9. You'll need a firm grip on the baby as it comes out because it will be slippery, so put on your Adam Gilchrist specials.

10. If you have got to this point you're our personal hero, but there is still a bit to go. Pass the baby to Mum's naked

belly and then cover the baby with a towel or blanket to keep it warm.

11. Don't touch the umbilical cord unless it's wrapped around the baby's neck.

12. By now you should either have medical care in the room with you or medical professionals on the phone with you.

13. RELAX, the baby's out. Enjoy the moment, book the PR agency, start writing your memoirs, make sure Mum's awake and don't forget that the placenta will be coming out soon. When it has come out, you can cut the umbilical cord.

Chapter 8

Birth

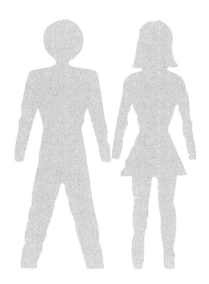

FOR H♀R

It doesn't matter whether you're going to give birth in a hospital, birthing centre, pool at home or in the back of your car, birth is your introduction to the world of parenting in more ways than one.

Most obviously, you actually get to see your bambino for the first time and it cements your position in history as a parent. You'll probably even replace your Facebook profile photo with a photo of your baby. It's serious stuff. On another front, you're about to find out just how opinionated and competitive the world of parenting is. When it comes to kids, people have very strong opinions on what is right and wrong. When we say 'strong' opinions, we're not sure that is a strong enough word. The birth place, who will catch your baby, pain medication, natural or Caesarean, birth techniques—you'll get different points of view from everyone you talk to. Once the baby comes you'll face the same problem when it comes to breastfeeding, circumcision, child care, nutrition, education and just about every facet of raising your kids. People like to believe what they did, or are doing, is the right way and everything else is pretty close to negligence. If you take it seriously, it can really mess with your head.

Our advice is to listen intently, smile and nod politely, then forget everything you heard and move on. Being a parent is intuitive; it pays to listen to your intuition and do what's best for you. What works for your mates may not work for you, so be open minded and willing to try new things. Being super set in your ways before the baby comes out can make the whole parenting caper bloody stressful. It pays to have a plan but one that is flexible!

Many guys are under the false impression that their partner knows exactly what to do when it comes to birthing and parenting. That's often not the case, and it can result in more pressure for you and an excuse for him to do bugger all. You need to be wary of the 'whatever you want, darling' approach.

Understanding your birthing options empowers the two of you to make a more informed decision and to get a better feeling for what is really right for you both. Even if you start out with your mind set on a specific birthing option, have you both really looked into what other options are available to you? It may not result in you changing your mind but it will make you both think more thoroughly about what you do and don't want from your birth. Films such as *The Business of Being Born* by Ricki Lake and *Orgasmic Birth* by Debra Pascali-Bonaro are worth watching, because both challenge the modern norm of childbirth.

Researching this book and making our films required us to take a look (for the first time) at water births, home births, birthing centres and everything in between. What we learned is that there is no right and wrong way to give birth, but there probably is a right way for you and your partner. Exploring all the options makes sense. You wouldn't buy a new car without looking at a few makes and models and weighing up their features and benefits. You would talk to friends, family and experts. Having a baby is a bit more important than buying a car, so we should all explore birthing options in detail just to see what's out there. And remember, it's just like buying a car in that you'll run into passionate and biased sales people. Just make sure you bring your own judgement to the picture.

Getting him to look into birthing options can be as difficult as getting him to go shopping for new curtains. In this chapter we will give him some food for thought on the birthing caper. We aim to walk the highwire between information overload and piquing his curiosity. One thing you can do is write a list of people you both know and put down how they gave birth. Also, talk to other couples about their experience. Also, give him a list of guys to talk to.

Labour and birth will be easier if you're more relaxed. Leaving the family home and entering a hospital can be stressful for some, but having a baby at home away from the perceived safety of a hospital is stressful for others. What's right for you? What's right for him?

Being a bloke at birth

Birth is best described as an emasculating event for a man. Everything is effectively out of his hands and into yours, the baby catcher's and the gods'. It's the ultimate nightmare for the fixer/problem solver. Watching your partner in pain (even when it's a natural and healthy pain) is not enjoyable. When your children get sick there will be times when you will just wish you could magically take on their illness, leaving them healthy and pain free. At some time during the birth he will feel like this. Being a bystander watching your pain is no fun. He loves and cares for you and he'll want your pain to go away and for everyone to be healthy and happy, and he will feel there's pretty close to sweet FA he can do about it. We'll show him what he can do to help you with your pain, how to be supportive and what NOT to say during the delivery.

As you approach birth you may have all sorts of Hollywood stereotypes in mind as to how it will proceed. One of the biggest stereotypes is women screaming at their partner, blaming them for putting them in the position of immense pain and discomfort. Having interviewed hundreds of dads across the world we're yet to meet one whose wife actually screamed at them. That being said, we're certain most women want their partners to be informed about birth should they need to make important decisions. You'd probably also like him to know how to help you and how not to annoy you—that's where we come in.

The birth of your child should be an amazing day. It may well be the greatest emotional moment that two people can share. We know that the birth is about you, that you're doing all of the work and that it's not exactly a walk in the park. What about him, though? We would like to think it can be an amazing day for him too, especially if he is calm, knows what's happening, feels he has some control and can provide the type of support you need.

The history of dads and birth

In the past men haven't really been welcome at, invited to or expected to be at birth. Different cultures have required fathers to do all sorts of things, including standing at the door of the birth hut with a spear as protection, cutting himself with animal teeth to simulate the pain of childbirth and being banished from the village altogether. Throughout time, even in western cultures, men have been forbidden to be present at births. One poor German doctor who was so desperate to witness a birth in the 1600s dressed as a woman and entered a birth chamber. Unfortunately, he was soon caught out by one of the midwives. His punishment? He was burnt to death with fellow physicians looking on.

Even in the 1960s and 1970s it was tough for guys to be present at the birth; some dads resorted to handcuffing themselves to their partners! We're sure there is a percentage of today's men who'd rather cut themselves to shreds with a lion's tooth than attend the birth, but they are rare. We feel sorry for men who miss the birth of their children for three reasons:

1. They miss out on witnessing a personal miracle and the most spiritual or moving moment of their life.

2. They suffer the anxiety of sitting around not knowing what is going on with the health of their partner and child for hours, even days. It would be unbearable.

3. They get a true understanding of just how strong women are. Most men never forget that, regardless of what happens in the marriage or in the rest of their life.

Fortunately, dads are now considered an important part of the birthing process. Different guys want to play different roles. To use a sporting analogy, we would describe them as coach, player or spectator. What does he want to be and what would you like him to be? Where are you having the baby and who else will be present to help you both through the process?

His role at the birth

Exactly what he will do will be at least partly dictated by what he's comfortable with. Some guys just don't want to be down the members' end when the baby is coming out. It can be because they are squeamish at the site of blood and bodily excretions, or it can be that they are worried that if they see a baby emerge from you it may cause irreparable damage to the way they see you sexually. Both are valid.

Although it is hard to believe, it is possible that some men can find sex post-birth difficult because they were traumatised by the image of the birth. Also, we've heard many women say they didn't want their partner to watch their bits stretch and contort. We haven't found any studies about this, but it does warrant discussion before the birth. Talk about what makes you both comfortable and respect each other's feelings.

There are three major options for him being in the birth room.

The coach

The coach is the sort of guy who needs to feel he has some control over every situation. He knows (or thinks he knows) what's going on, isn't afraid to ask questions of the doctor or midwife and is keen to talk you through the birth with positive reinforcement. He'll be proactive, interactive, have no fear of the members' end . . . and quite annoying if that's not what you're after.

The team-mate

He's focused on you and your needs. He's attentive, supportive and trying to juggle what you want and what the baby catchers are saying. He knows the game plan and will try to help you make it happen. He's prepared to listen to you and the baby catchers and step in to make a hard decision if need be, but that will take a great deal of courage.

The spectator

He'll be unflinchingly up your end of the table, holding your hand and trying his best to be positive and comforting for you while largely staring at his feet. He may not be comfortable participating actively or engaging with the baby catchers.

Which one of these will your partner be? Which one would you like him to be?

What emotions will he experience during birth?

Concern and fear

It doesn't matter what role he plays or how positive and confident he is, he will be worrying about you both A LOT. If he's not well prepared for birth and doesn't have a good understanding of what will happen (and can happen) his anxiety will be greater. Let's not forget there is still a chance he's in a Neanderthal-like state of denial and his reaction may be sheer surprise: Wow, it's a baby in there! Who'd have thought!

What to do about pain—alleviate or eradicate?

Since the dawn of time women have feared the pain of birth (and rightly so). Different cultures have had their own versions of pain relief, including opium, coca leaves, hypnotism and cassowary anus. Some tribes also believed eating eels would make the birth canal slippery and the birth therefore easier. It's interesting that women seem to have tried to alleviate pain and men have tried to eradicate it.

If you look back at the origins of modern pain medication you'll see it was male doctors who are to blame, or thank depending on your view. Once male doctors came on the birth scene they found it difficult to witness the pain of birth. Being fixers and problem solvers they sought ways of eradicating pain altogether. We'd like to think their efforts had women's best interests at heart but it's conceivable that it was more to relieve their own 'pain' as they watched and listened to women in labour.

Today's man shares the same philosophy. We'd have taken a slug on the gas if they had offered it to us and many guys would happily recommend their partner opt for pain eradication after seeing them in pain for a few hours (or even minutes). It's no fun for him.

If your plan is to have a natural and drug-free birth, make sure he knows if and when it's OK to call for pain relief and when you need him to be strong and supportive and help you through the pain. We'll arm him with some natural pain relief techniques that can help you in his section of this chapter.

Complete respect

Just about every guy we interviewed said that during birth they felt utter respect and love for their partner and her ability to get through labour and get the baby out. Every man who has witnessed a birth will forever respect women for their ability to cope with pain.

Sheer joy

When the baby is out and you're both well he will feel an unrivalled sense of joy and happiness. That moment is one of sheer relief, amazement and happiness. Many men say that the day their first child was born was the most amazing moment in their life.

Physical and emotional exhaustion

It's difficult to believe that birth can be exhausting for men, but it's true. He's likely to be just as tired as you are leading into the birth, and a long labour is physically and mentally taxing even though you're doing all the work. Nothing can really prepare him for how physically and emotionally draining his first birth experience will be.

What can he do for you during birth?

Keep you fed and watered

Despite the fact that you probably feel as if you have already run a marathon, haven't slept properly in weeks and haven't had an alcoholic beverage in months, staying hydrated and keeping your energy levels up is imperative. In terms of energy expended, birth has been likened to a brisk 6 kilometre walk. We know, the analogy seems ridiculous: at nine months you're no more capable of going for a brisk walk than you are of doing a graceful half pike off the 10 metre diving platform at your local swimming pool. During this particular 'brisk walk' it's his job to make sure you drink lots of water and eat something that will give you energy. It's an intense workout and your mind isn't going to be on Gatorade and bananas.

From his perspective it's great too, because it gives him something to focus on and do even if he's never felt less like John Wayne in his life. He needs distractions to keep his brain from thinking too much. Only minutes of self-denial remain . . .

Help you stay calm and relaxed

For most women, it can be disconcerting having people walking in and out of your birthing room. Our furry friends in the animal kingdom can totally stop their contractions if they are startled or concerned about a change in their physical environment, but those of us with a big brain cannot, alas.

There can be people (midwives, nurses, obstetricians, even occasionally medical students) looking at foetal monitors, taking blood pressure, checking your dilation and a million other distractions. Even when it's just the two of you there may be moments when you doubt your ability to get through the birth, or just feel anxiety and fear.

We know from the men we've spoken to that your partner will be feeling that he is contributing nothing, but we also know that having him there at the birth will probably reduce your stress.

Be aware that this is not really your day: the baby is a very active participant in the birth. The day's activities are actually happening largely at your baby's discretion. Our best advice here is to trust in nature. This is a natural, normal event that has been happening amazingly successfully for millions of years. As things heat up, and nerves, contraction and birth starts to settle in, reassuring, calm and supportive behaviours become more and more important.

From this perspective, there are several things you can do to help everyone out.

Help you be as comfortable as possible

Comfort is relative, and the truth is no matter what he does or how well he does it, birth is going to involve pain. But although things like hot packs, cold packs, extra pillows, a wet flannel, a massage or foot rub or running you a bath may seem totally inadequate, they actually can help.

By helping out and understanding something about the process he'll be keeping occupied, feeling valuable and having a better experience.

Help you change birthing positions

You're not exactly going to be super mobile, so you may need his help to get into various positions. Once again, involving him will help you and make him feel he is a part of the birth. Think of birthing positions in terms of *Dancing with the Stars*: you wouldn't go on the show and not practise beforehand. You'd want to make sure that when Tom the Chippy's shirt comes off you don't go to water on national TV. Same goes with birth positions. Make sure he knows what they are and how to do them so he's not a bumbling fool who will score a series of 0 out of 10s from you, the judge.

On another note, many of the birth positions you may adopt on the day require quite some strength. Most blokes think exercising anything south of the border is a complete waste of time; we like the glamour muscles of the upper body. Squatting during birth with all that weight cannot be easy, so practise beforehand so that your muscles, and his, have time to build up strength.

Provide emotional support by saying the right things

It's not easy to know what to say when your partner is uncomfortable, in pain or in need of support. We'll arm him with plenty of positive things to help you along and give him some good advice on what not to say!

*   *   *

We hope we've established that he can play an active role in the birth that will be beneficial to you. Talk to him about what you would like him to do so that he can be prepared going into the birth.

We wish you all the very best for your birth experience. If you're both prepared—which, given you are reading this book, is highly likely—then you've done everything you can to maximise the chances of having a happy and enjoyable experience together.

This is it, your last few days as a family of two. Take some time to think about the change in dynamics in your relationship once the baby arrives. Remember that you will be very focused on the baby in the next six months or more, but try to remember that your man also needs some of your love and attention. By making a joint effort to keep a healthy relationship a high priority you will make the first year of parenting easier and keep your relationship strong and happy. What's the point of going through all that you have just done if you have a crappy relationship at the end?

If you want a first-hand account of what is going through a man's mind during labour and birth, flick to page 204 for Troy's Birth Blog.

FOR HIM

The births of your children should be among the most memorable days of your life but it can be genuinely frightening, confronting, difficult and mentally exhausting. It's a day that lends itself to the unprepared bloke going into sub-cranium meltdown. But think about this for a second: a bloke who is having his second baby, even years after his first, is a model of coolness. Why? He's had some experience and knows what to expect. If you can get your head around what you're in for, you'll take some of the edge off the experience, be more helpful and enjoy it more. We know from our experiences.

The birth of our first babies were panics. Even though, objectively, everything was pretty close to smooth sailing, on the inside of our heads we were lurching from one panicky moment to the next. They were harrowing days, mainly because we had little idea what was happening, why it was happening or what our roles were.

When our babies were born, we were frazzled. We were so relieved that no one's head fell off, all we wanted to do was celebrate for 30 minutes and then hibernate for a few months to recover. We guess it was a bit like a flight from London to Sydney where you don't sleep a single wink and are worried the whole time that the wings are about to fall off the plane. The bad part of this is that we actually missed the whole experience. We were so stressed and wide-eyed that nothing remained in our craniums for longer than five seconds.

The really tough part of the 'she'll be right, mate' approach is that when the baby is born there is no hibernation. There isn't even any time for much rest. The adrenaline gives way to severe tiredness. It's a bit like the way all of this started: a massive moment of relief, happiness, contentment, but then on with life, the job. The best thing, for everyone, is to get to the starting line with you, your partner and your new baby as peaceful, relaxed and rested as possible and, honestly, you can have a huge impact on that. By 'starting line' we mean the moment when you stand unbelievably proud of your partner and with your baby in your arms.

Finish reading this paragraph, then put the book down for a minute. Try to picture yourself holding a little baby wrapped up in a blanket. You're in a hospital room, cradling a baby, your baby. Seriously, no one is watching you . . . Close your eyes and picture it. It's going to happen. And soon.

Here's the point. Our second babies' births were much more relaxed. For everyone. It was like arriving again at Sydney airport but this time having flown first class, had a seriously solid sleep and ready to hit the ground running for a full day of sightseeing and enjoyment. We had confidence that everything was going to be OK. We knew the wings weren't going to fall off. We knew our role, we knew what was happening, we knew the layout of the room.

And what was the difference between economy class frazzled and first class cool? Our brains. Our preparedness. Our ability to know our place and to be cool, supportive and trusting in nature and our wives. Believe us, women know what do to. Their gender is tougher, stronger and more brilliant than ours. Let her do her thing.

Be the first-class fella.

Keep that mental image of you with the baby close. During the birth, every minute, every contraction is taking you closer to that reality. The cooler and smoother you are the better you'll be at the starting line. So let's get on with it.

By now you've decided (hopefully) where to have the baby and who will be present. You'll have familiarised yourself with the place and the people, know what should happen and what could happen and have some sort of birth plan. If you haven't, bring it up with your partner.

In sporting terms birth is the grand final of pregnancy, but in parenting terms it's a second-round game of a lifelong season. Just like the AFL, NRL or the A League, birth really is a team event. It's easy to think that the birth is out of your hands, that you are just a paying spectator, but to get the most out of the event and to have the best possible experience you need to be well prepared.

What role will you play at the birth? What can you do to be an active participant, to make your partner more relaxed and comfortable and to make the experience the best possible one for you?

The history of blokes and birth

Birth has long been the domain of women only. It didn't matter whether you belonged to a tribe in Africa, had a hand in building the great pyramids or lived in Europe in the 1800s, chances are you wouldn't have been present at the birth.

Men attending birth is a recent phenomenon and we can all thank a guy called Robert Bradley for our ability to do so. Bradley was known as the father of fathers. He presided over 21,000 unmedicated births and published a book titled *Fathers' Presence in the Delivery Room* in 1962. He studied what happened when fathers were present during labour and concluded that we actually help our partners relax and we reduce anxiety.

In Europe in the 1600s men were forbidden in the birth chamber. One German physician was reportedly so desperate to witness a birth that he dressed as a woman and tried to pass himself off as a midwife. Sometime later male doctors started seeing an opportunity to make money out of birthing. Midwives were starting to be paid for their services by the wealthy, and the men of the day didn't want to miss out on the action. Early obstetricians were known as barber surgeons, and they set about discrediting the role played by midwives. Over the next few hundred years this constant attacking just about made the art of midwifery extinct.

Men took a natural process, tried to make it easier and in the process completely stuffed it up. We developed forceps and suction cups, tried to eradicate pain through drugs and generally tried to reinvent the entire birthing process. It's no wonder women have tried to keep us out of the birthing caper for so long; they knew we would completely balls it up and they were pretty spot on.

Since the dawn of time women have tried to ease the pain of childbirth through natural means. Some of these efforts certainly seem a little hippie-ish: who would fancy eating cassowary anus, eating eels to make the birth canal slippery or munching on coca leaves? Interestingly, we could find ZERO examples of women trying to eradicate the pain of childbirth altogether. When male doctors first witnessed the pain of childbirth they found it unbearable and barbaric and set about finding ways to make birth faster, easier and painless. There's nothing like a short cut! Our wives were VERY up for the male way of doing things, though, so it's not all bad. At least now we have a choice about pain relief in pregnancy.

We are the first generation who is expected to be at the birth. What role are we expected to play, can we play, should we play or do we want to play?

Some interesting facts around birth

- The term 'gossip' originated when women who assisted at births were termed gossips. (Why?)
- Barber surgeons dressed as women in the early days in an effort to make the women more relaxed. Bearded men in dresses make us nervous.
- The doctor who first developed the epidural tested it on his assistant by injecting him, then pulling out his pubic hair, squeezing his testicle and burning him to see if he could feel any pain. Let's hope the assistant got overtime for that assignment!
- You may have heard of Lamaze classes. Old Dr Lamaze was so appalled at witnessing the pain experienced during birth that he spent the duration of his first child's birth getting pole-axed at the local bar. He did a better job at subsequent births and a great job of keeping that nugget of information off the front cover of the March 1962 edition of *Who Weekly*!

More labour than a working bee at Julia Gillard's house: lights, camera, contraction

The song 'Final Countdown' by Queen should be a part of your birth mix and at this point it's worth dialling the volume up to ten. This, our friend, is the final countdown indeed. Here are four signs that your partner is in labour:

1. *Bloody show.* Sounds like something our dads would have yelled at the TV during a bad episode of *Hey Hey, It's Saturday*, but in birth terms it is a red or pinkish discharge that may suggest that dilation of the cervix has started. It may be accompanied by a mucous plug—there's that word

again. The mucous plug at the opening of the uterus keeps all the nasties (like you) out during pregnancy.

2. *Contractions.* As contractions get stronger and closer together it's a good sign that things are happening. Beware of Braxton-Hicks, which are something akin to your partner's body having practice contractions. They're also good at scaring the shit out of you both. Keep a captain's log of the length of time of the contractions and the time gap between them (from the start of one till the start of the next). The longer, stronger and closer together they are the closer you are to becoming a dad! Your sphincter may start contracting of its own accord, and your nerves will be starting to jangle!!

3. *Back and thigh ache (hers, not yours), if it persists.*

4. *Water 'breaks'/releases.* It might be a trickle or a gush. Only 10–15 per cent of women experience this before going into labour.

It's really important to remember that the symptoms don't follow any obvious, predetermined path. As noted above, for instance, there may not be any 'breaking' of the waters at all. The best bet is to listen to your partner and follow her cues. Have your hospital plans prepared and bags packed and be ready to go over the trenches at any time!

When the contractions start your first reaction will be to throw the bags in the car and speed off to the hospital, but if she isn't ready they will send you right back home. The tough part of early labour is there is no guarantee as to how long it will take before you need to get mobile or at least call in the baby catchers. You both have to know the signs and listen to what her body is telling her, then you can make a judgement call. If either of you is in doubt, call your baby catchers or the hospital and talk them through the symptoms.

Call the baby-catching team:

- When she experiences contractions lasting one minute each and coming every five minutes or less. We've come across blokes who've plotted contractions on spreadsheets—it's not necessary, but it might help you take your mind off what's about to happen.

- If water releases ('breaks'). Look at the colour of the discharge and let your caregiver know if either of you notice anything unusual—green, brown or black colour, say. Personally, we consider a litre of amniotic fluid appearing on the carpet 'unusual', but as with everything in pregnancy you need to completely rethink the word 'unusual'.

- If there's heavy vaginal bleeding, constant abdominal pain or fever above 37.2°C.

- If she has contractions before 37 weeks.

- If she has persistent headaches, intense pain or tenderness.

- If something doesn't feel right. Sometimes mums can just feel that something isn't right. If she is concerned or feeling unwell, contact your caregiver.

It's worth repeating: your job is to stay calm and be reassuring. If things start kicking off in the middle of the night don't roll over and go back to sleep—start being her birth partner and getting excited that your baby is on its way.

A layman's guide to the three stages of birth

Stage 1: Dilation (the gates are open!)

Ina May Gaskin, a world-famous midwife, is famous for the saying, 'She is going to get huge!' We only wish she had said it with an Arnold Schwarzenegger accent. As Ina aptly reminds us, when us blokes get excited blood rushes straight to the penis, it swells and . . . gets huge. (God love you, Ina—that's the first time anyone has said that to us!)

In almost exactly the same way, during birth blood rushes to your partner's vagina. It swells, then opens for the baby and 'gets huge'. It's meant to do that. It takes a while, but it is a big part of the process of birth. Without a lot of back story it's probably not a great idea to encourage her to get huge, but baffling her with some Arnie encouragement might just take the edge off a few contractions!

As younger, more naive fellows we thought the painful part (you know, the bits where Hollywood shows the screaming and physical abuse of husbands) was as the baby stretched the vagina on its final step out into the world. We assumed the pain was at its maximum when the widest part of the head was half in and half out, so to speak. Not so.

Stage 1 is separated into three phases of dilation:

1. early (0–3 centimetres)
2. active (4–7 centimetres)
3. transition (8–10 centimetres)

During labour, the cervix (the opening of the uterus) dilates because the uterus, which is a very large muscle, tightens and contracts. This happens on and off for many hours, and in later stages of labour the sensations (contractions, waves, surges . . . there are many words used to describe them) gradually increase in length, strength and number until the cervix is fully dilated, to about 10 centimetres.

Early labour—ready, steady . . .

There's no exact guide, but early stage contractions can last for six to twelve hours (or longer). Try to get your partner to rest and stay hydrated—it may be a long day or night ahead.

We regularly hear that a woman will wake up her partner and say, 'I've been having contractions for a few hours now.' In early labour, she can pretty much talk through contractions and describe them to you (and smile between them). You'll know when the contractions are getting more regular and painful. There's no need to break out the stopwatch just yet, coach!

Early labour catchwords

'Encourage', 'stay calm', 'enjoy' and 'rest'.

Now is the time to start being super awesome. Although neither of you has much say in the process, the longer you can hang out at this stage without losing much energy or stress the better everyone will be. Here are seven ways to help both of you do that:

1. Watch movies.
2. Listen to her favourite music.
3. Read to her or get her something to read.
4. Take a bath or shower (together might be nice).
5. Give her a massage.
6. Find your birth plan and review it together.
7. Just be there to enjoy the excitement of what is about to happen.

Everyone's pain thresholds are different, so the best bet is to listen intently and calmly to your partner and do what you can to work out where you are in the process.

Why does it hurt? At full term, the uterus is the biggest muscle in her body. It contracts on autopilot and when it does it restricts blood flow to the muscles and stops waste being removed. The build-up causes burning and pain and the muscle contractions are like severe cramp (if you've ever had one you'd appreciate it). Pelvic ligaments get stretched, Fallopian tubes and ovaries are pulled and the baby's head and spine may scrape across her back. Its head compresses the bowels and bladder.

Rejoice in your lack of a uterus. This, our friends, is a job for the ladies.

Active labour—the umpire has blown his whistle and it's game on

This is where the cervix dilates to 4–7 centimetres. Active labour, on average, is shorter (four to six hours) than early labour. Contractions will be more uncomfortable. If she can't talk normally any more and is really working hard to cope, those are good signs that it's all getting close. Don't tell her you're glad she can't talk and it's a good sign. During labour, when a thought comes into your head, just mull it over for a few seconds before blurting it out. You'll never be more likely to say things that can be misinterpreted or taken badly.

Use the pain management techniques listed on pages 197 and 202 and offer words of encouragement and support. If you're not already there, active labour is when you should go to the hospital or birth centre.

Five signs that she's doing well in labour

1. She can relax her shoulders and jaw during a contraction.
2. She vomits (yes, throwing up is actually a good sign).
3. She moves her body in a rhythmic motion during contractions (much like Michael Jackson rap dancing minus the moonwalking).
4. She's relaxed during contractions.
5. She can still smile between contractions or she falls asleep between them. Resting between contractions is a really important skill. She's saving energy for the labour ahead.

Transition—it's not called labour for nothing!

During transition the cervix fully dilates to 7–10 centimetres. This is the hardest part of labour, but it's also the shortest: it usually lasts less than two hours. This is the part of labour that can knock the unprepared bloke for six. There is a point in the labour where your partner will change gears; she will stop being chatty and get quiet, introverted and focused on the job ahead. She may talk about not being able to do it, about needing drugs or about going home for a while and coming back next week. Or she may look like Steve Waugh coming out to bat with Australia at four for bugger all and needing plenty.

Your unprepared bloke may take this quietness as weakness and jump in with a choreographed routine of support. Top marks for effort, mate, but wrong time. This quietness is an important and very normal stage of progress, and signals the beginning of the last stage. This is usually when the cowboy gets sent away to start boiling the water. Let her have her time to focus. Now is the time to 'just be there'. If you pick this, you are a hero. It's also an awesome time to contemplate what the next few hours will bring. After nine months, cravings, worry, stress, hormones and the whole box and dice, this is it. Take a minute to smell the roses, watch your partner and marvel at the oncoming experience.

- She may go into a zone or ask for drugs.
- She may need your intense support at this time or she may snap and yell at you. If she says 'Don't touch me', it's a great indication that she's in transition.
- She may vomit. That's another great sign that things are moving along. This may be the only time that vomiting is a sign of a good thing . . . for most of us vomiting is usually bought on by drinking too much or eating something dodgy or waking up with a member of Savage Garden in your bed—nothing positive there!
- She may start to feel rectal pressure. What? Yep. The baby's head has to pass by the colon and rectum before it gets to the vagina, so she actually feels like she needs to 'drop the kids off at the pool' and in fact she may well do so. Romantic, no. The truth and completely natural, yes. She's probably fairly stressed about snapping off in front of you and the hospital staff, and there's no need to remind her of it EVER. If it were us, we'd have touched cloth well before the baby got into the same postcode as our colons through fear alone!

Stage 2: Pushing and birth

Put on some energetic music at this point and bring out the lemon essential oil to wake up the room! It's time for the big arrival! Maybe you have a prearranged birth song or a maternity mix on the iPod you'd like the baby to come out to. Here are a few suggested tracks:

- 'Under Pressure', Queen
- 'Push It', Salt-n-Pepa

- 'Welcome to the Jungle', Guns 'n' Roses
- 'Anybody Seen My Baby?', Rolling Stones
- 'My Name Is', Eminem
- 'Stronger', Kanye West (purely for the lyrics 'I need you to hurry up now, cos I can't wait much longer').

Just some suggestions. Feel free to choose your own.

Unless your doctor or midwife tells her otherwise, the best times to start pushing are when she feels the need to push or her body just does it without thinking about it. Ideally the head will have already passed down through the cervix and pressed against your partner's pelvic floor muscles. This is where all those Kegel exercises will be paying off.

By this time you're likely to have a midwife, doula or caregiver with you to help guide your baby out. The gates are open, the tunnel is wide enough (well, it ain't getting any wider) and the world beckons for your nipper. You may well choose to stay up at the northern end of the arena at this stage. There are no prizes for staying down the members' end if it makes you feel uncomfortable or for peeking over the curtain during a Caesarean. Do what feels right and support your partner. She needs you now.

The baby is now making its way down the birth canal. As the uterus contracts and relaxes the baby inches forward, then back. Different birthing positions and paraphernalia (see page 198) may be needed to help her feel as comfortable as possible.

TROY: With the birth of my second baby, the obstetrician suggested trying stirrups and handles. He reacted to the look of confusion/disbelief on our faces and gave a brief and almost incomprehensible talk about African women and how their hips and pelvises work, and thought it worth a try. So try it we did. Almost like magic, the wheels started to spin, we started to get some traction and we were in business. This goes against the grain of everything we'd learned but just goes to show that keeping an open mind and trying different positions can help. It will probably attract the ire of every midwife and doula on the planet and for that I'm sorry . . . when Stacey gave birth on her back in *Being Dad* 1 I was almost run out of every town the film was shown in.

At this stage, although it's just about impossible to work out what's going on, keep an eye out for the top of the baby's head and keep on being supportive. Once the little tufts of hair attached to a squishy pale-looking lemon became distinguishable the 'denial button' stops working. There's really a baby en route! And it's mine!!

NO ONE TOLD ME WE WERE HAVING A BABY HERE!!! Oh yeah, that's right . . . they've been saying that for a few months now.

Freeze frame. Now, the panicky bloke in this position is living a very uncomfortable dual experience: 95 per cent of his brain is desperately keen for the contractions and birth experience to be safely over and the baby to be here. The remaining 5 per cent of his brain is feeling very unsure whether he will be a good dad for the rest of his life. He's thinking, *I'm not ready for this, I'm not ready for this, I'm not ready for this.*

> TROY: Although she initially resisted the idea, my wife found it very helpful to have a mirror strategically held up so that she could see what type of pushing was working. For her, the combo of the stirrups, handles and mirror was just the tonic. As she got the visual hang of what was working and what wasn't, things sped up immeasurably. Getting the third year medical student to hold the mirror straight was no easy task. The poor bloke was staring straight at the gates of Troy, attending his first birth and his hands were shaking so badly I could see my own reflection in the mirror. Bloody amateurs. I didn't offer to take over though . . . the kid had to learn somehow right?

Hold her hand, mop her brow, and get her a drink or some crushed ice. Tell her she's doing great and that you love her. If you're down the members' end you'll soon understand the full extent of the obstetricians' phrase 'elasticity of the vagina'.

Warning—the episiotomy!

We have had lots of delightful feedback from our *Being Dad* films. In fact, we have received major pieces of gratitude in relation to two specific events in the birth. One of them is knowing what an episiotomy is, when it's about to happen and when to look away.

Despite the natural elasticity of the vagina, pressure being applied from the emerging baby may start to become too much for the surrounding skin to deal with. In the event it gets too much the skin between the vagina and the anus (the perineum) can actually tear, ultimately allowing the extra little bit of wiggle room that the baby may need. Rather than allow the skin to tear, which can be difficult, painful and messy, the obstetrician may call for a set of scissors to aid proceedings.

If you can avoid this particular visual experience our advice is to do so. It is a very important, valuable medical practice and your partner is unlikely to even know that it has happened. But does any man really need to see his partner's vagina cut with a pair of scissors? We both know the answer to that one.

The moral of this story is if you see a pair of scissors at any stage, look the other way. It only takes a second, seems to work well and your partner will barely seem to notice.

When the scissors go away, you can go back to business.

The pushing stage can last from anywhere from several minutes to several hours.

Birth is one of the world's great events you can watch live, from spotting the scalp and hair to holding your baby. Very few moments cause the world to stand still the way it does when your baby emerges. You don't breathe. You don't move. You probably won't blink for three or four minutes, and you may even be speechless for the first time in your life!

One can only imagine the feeling from a woman's perspective— the release and relaxation must be a thousand times greater. It's as if in an instant she goes from maximum pain to maximum pleasure—it seems holding the baby is the greatest painkiller of all!

Much like the conclusion of the conception stage, the climax of the pregnancy is a huge release. Love, and outpouring of emotion, fluids and plenty of other stuff! Expect to cry; don't hold back.

Natural pain management techniques

As we've already suggested, blokes have a history of not coping well with watching women giving birth. It seems our pain threshold is significantly lower than theirs even when it's them in pain! When labour kicks in you'll be more than ready to throw the birth plan that called for a natural, drug-free birth into the bin and start signalling to the sidelines for the magic spray and the best epidural money can buy.

If you've made the decision to opt for a natural birth, a few pain management techniques should be part of your plan. Labour and birth happen best when mothers feel supported and respected and allowed to do what feels natural to them. Much of labour is literally in her head (again, DEFINITELY SOMETHING NOT TO SAY OUT LOUD)—her brain produces hormones that stimulate contractions and how she copes with labour depends on her brain making hormones called oxytocin and endorphins.

Support and encouragement have a huge influence on how well she can surrender during labour and feel confident that she can open herself to have her baby with her own power. This is where you, as her birth partner, can be a source of support and encouragement to her.

This isn't to say that every woman can have a medication-free birth. No matter how tough your partner is or how many babies she's had, there may be times when medication is needed. Your job isn't to judge, it's to encourage and support her and to know when it's OK to deviate from what you had planned to what's needed. The only thing you can do to minimise your anxiety is be prepared, and talk about these possibilities together before labour.

If you planned to use an epidural to deal with labour pain she'll still have several hours of labour to deal with before she can get that awfully large needle in the back, so practising pain management techniques using different methods and different positions is going to be important. Don't be afraid to stick a few Post-its onto important pages of your plan or whatever book you're using and take it into the delivery room.

There are many great natural ways of increasing the body's ability to give birth easily, and they have been used throughout the ages. We would probably just go straight for the good stuff, but we should consider these.

Natural childbirth is not about suffering. Misery in childbirth is not acceptable, so if she gets to a point where she's suffering and not coping well it's time to opt for pain medication. Remember, even the best birth plan may need to be thrown out. No one gets a medal for how much pain they put up with.

Women who want to have a natural childbirth have a right to be supported to do that. You're very important in supporting her wishes.

Making birth easier by changing positions during labour and while pushing
Like just about every modern bloke you probably thought, before you did your birth plan at least, that she'd be giving birth on her

back, the way we've all seen so much on TV and in the movies. Well, now you know better. It's often not comfortable for most women to be on their back during labour for more than a few minutes or a few pushes here and there. They rarely choose this position when given a choice. Here are a few pros and cons of different birthing positions you might consider and try:

- *Standing*
  Pros: Excellent for using gravity, reducing pain and speeding up labour.
  Cons: Can make it difficult for the doctor or midwife to control proceedings and catch the baby.

TIP

Stand over a clean, soft surface!!

- *Walking*
  Pros: Uses gravity, can reduce pain and speed up delivery. Handy if walking to the hospital if you run out of petrol.
  Cons: Not appropriate if mum has high blood pressure and not possible if she has had an epidural. Also, it's tough to catch the baby from a mobile mum.

- *Sitting*
  Pros: Uses gravity, conserves energy and can help with the baby's descent.
  Cons: May not be appropriate if mum has high blood pressure. May stain the upholstery on the Jason recliner.

- *Using a birth ball*
  Pros: More comfortable on Mum's behind and perineum. It can help relax the pelvis and is great for resting her arms and head on.

Cons: Your partner may feel unbalanced sitting on it and it can be harder for medical staff to monitor the baby when she is on the ball. You try balancing on a birth ball with a four kilogram medicine ball emerging from the orifice of your choice!

- *Sitting on a toilet*
  Pros: Uses gravity, and subconsciously she's used to letting go there.
  Cons: It's not the most attractive environment, and she may find it causes too much pressure on her perineum.

- *Semi-sitting*
  Pros: Comfortable, uses gravity and is good for letting the doctor, midwife or you see what's going on.
  Cons: Limits mobility of sacrum (the back of the pelvis), which decreases the space in the pelvis for the baby.

- *On the back with legs raised*
  Pros: Doctor, midwife and nurse can see well and can help get baby under the pubic bone.
  Cons: Requires your partner to push the baby against gravity (literally up towards the ceiling), is generally uncomfortable, increases perineal tears and increases usage of tools and incisions for birth.

- *Side-lying*
  Pros: Provides many benefits, including a good resting position for mum, speeding up labour and a lower risk of tearing. You'll need to support her leg in this position.
  Cons: Can feel awkward for mum, and her hips can become sore if she's on one side too long. Having to hold up her leg for extended periods of time is exhausting.

- *Leaning against you or a wall*
  Pros: Promotes better, less painful contractions and can relieve backache.
  Cons: Can be tiresome on her legs (and yours!).

- *Kneeling*
  Pros: Good for use with a birth ball, encourages good positioning of the baby and reduces pressure in multiple areas.
  Cons: Can be hard on the knees and legs if done for long periods.

- *Squatting*
  Pros: Uses gravity, opens up pelvis and helps with baby rotation.
  Cons: Uncomfortable. See how you do squatting with a bowling ball for even five minutes!

- *On hands and knees*
  Pros: Good for back labour (where the baby is in a posterior position with the skull hard up against the pelvis), for turning a posterior baby or for big babies.
  Cons: Hard for mum to see what's going on. Also, some medical providers aren't used to catching babies in this position.

It's a pretty amazing set of combinations and permutations. As silly as it sounds, it really does pay to practise some of these moves in advance. It will help strengthen the muscles required to do them properly and will prepare you both for the big day.

Einstein's theory of gravity—how you can actually use it!
Gravity helps the birth process by:

- making contractions more effective and regular
- improving the dilation of the cervix

- improving your partner's ability to relax between contractions, and
- reducing the time of labour.

This all means a less painful labour.

If Einstein and Newton (who are considered the founders of the theory of gravity) were so smart, why didn't they tell us that babies are best born using gravity? We think it would have been far more useful than $E=mc^2$ and more productive than time spent making the atomic bomb. Perhaps if Newton had been hit on the head with a baby instead of an apple the world would be a different place.

We've reworked a few of their other theories:

1. Keep shooting small things up there and eventually something big will come back out.

2. For every one of your stupid actions you can expect a not so equal yet opposite reaction from your partner.

Other natural methods of relieving pain

You may think we've taken a slug on the pethidine and are wandering into the hippie world here, but below are nine natural pain-relieving techniques you can help with that may make things easier and better. They are well worth a look, and are definitely more worthwhile than the 'she'll-be-rightisms':

1. *Mental relaxation techniques.* These require practice in the months and weeks leading up to the birth. Taking a hypno birthing or a natural childbirth class enables you both to practise ways of mentally relaxing and letting go. If you attend such classes you will be awarded a medal of honour by the International Association of Fallopian Tubes.

2. *Physical comfort measures.* Hot and cold packs applied to areas of the body that are experiencing pain, discomfort or cramping can help a lot. Be sure to have these ready in

advance, but don't use them without asking her and don't insist on it. Don't use heat or cold on her if she has pain medication, though, because it could burn her or freeze her skin. Sipping warm tea or cool water can also help— it's your job to keep her hydrated. Hot and cold packs are a great gift idea before birth, but they aren't romantic, so maybe suggest them as a good pressie from the parents or your mates.

3. *Shower or bath.* During the early stage of labour many women find a shower or bath both relaxing and effective in reducing the discomfort of contractions. If you have a big tub at home, why not take a bath together? It may be the last time you can for a long time and it might even inspire some sex in early labour (a great thing!). What a memory! To be fair this was suggested by Jeanette, our doula friend. We don't think there would be many blokes who'd be looking for sex in the bath during labour—certainly not the can't do men among us. But if it sounds like a good idea, then tuck on in!

4. *Position changes.* Depending on how the baby is positioned and how the labour is progressing, trying some of the different positions mentioned earlier will most likely help with the delivery and reduce her discomfort. It's recommended that all mums try at least five positions more than once: walking, squatting, hands and knees, rocking on the birth ball and lying on the side. Practise these in advance, regularly, to help train her muscles to do them all with the extra weight of the baby.

5. *Mantras.* You both might want to chant—'Wiggle this baby out', 'Let your uterus do the work', 'Open' or whatever positive statement she thinks might help. Some mums call their baby's name. Others are very quiet. The key is for you to be calm, encourage her and remind her that this is all

good and the more she lets go the easier it will be. Chants that are not recommended include 'Hurry the f+ck up', 'Just come out of there you little shit' and 'Do you think he'll be out by the time the game starts?'

6. *Birth balls.* These are plastic's gift to pregnant women. Most women find them very helpful in pregnancy, amazingly helpful during labour and nice to bounce on with baby during the first year or so. Her level of interest in birth balls is likely to be inversely proportional to her interest in your balls—sounds like another theory we could sell to with the Royal Society of Physics Boffins.

7. *Squat bar.* Some hospitals have a bar that can attach to the hospital bed. Use it. Be creative! Actually, not that creative . . .

8. *Aromatherapy.* Smelling scents of essential oils such as lavender and peppermint can absolutely change the mood in a room and have a positive effect on your partner's hormone levels. Beer, cigarettes, BO and bad breath do not constitute scents that can have a positive effect on hormone levels, but they can certainly change the mood in a room (particularly one with a labouring woman).

9. *TENS (transcutaneous electrical nerve simulation).* A TENS unit is a clever electrical gizmo that stimulates the body's own natural painkillers with a small electric current that runs across mum's lower back and can be turned up or down as needed. It feels like a cat pawing her back. It's not commonly used in Australia but is available through physical therapy offices, and some doulas and childbirth educators know where to get the devices. We assume it's not to be used in conjunction with number three, above.

Hello, baby!

What's it really like in the trenches during delivery? In the *Being Dad* DVD Troy was filmed during the birth of his first baby, Matilda. It's one thing to watch him going through the process, but what was really going on in his head? Once the baby was born a dictaphone was thrust in his direction and he was asked to simply blurt out his thoughts, recollections and the things he learnt during the delivery. Here is what we could decipher from his post-birth state of delirium:

> People travel to all ends of the Earth searching for new sights and experiences. Not in my life have I ever witnessed anything like this before, though. It was quite an extraordinary sight to see the squished face of a baby literally stuck between my wife's legs. 'He' (as he later turned out to be a girl) was not breathing yet his whole face was out in the open. At this point the umbilical cord was still delivering all of the nutrients and oxygen that the baby needed to survive yet I was petrified that he wasn't able to breathe!
>
> During the pregnancy, the foetus has basically been underwater the whole time. Obviously it's not water, but you know what we mean. The baby has even been practising breathing by inhaling and expelling the fluid. When he or she comes out, the baby has got some drying out to do. You know what your fingertips are like if you linger in the pool or the surf for 30 minutes too long; that's what she looked like.
>
> I remember the smell, an almost raw, animal like smell of the baby, the amniotic fluid and all the other bits and pieces. Not offensive at all, just raw and earthy.
>
> I wasn't aware that mother's milk doesn't come in for a few days, to give the baby a chance to dry out. (Like the mobile phone technology Bluetooth, I've dubbed the miraculous communication between baby and boob 'boob-tooth'. The way

your missus' boobs communicate and respond to the baby is amazing . . . more later.)

At the immediate point, though, the baby's face is vertical so that the fluid can drain out of the airways. But at this unbelievable and very abstract juncture, my wife started to ever so slightly freak out. And understandably so. She had a baby half in and half out of her. Weird way to be. In fact, it was the one time in the whole process she kind of lost it for a second. It must be a weird sensation yet motivating to get the job completely done . . . ASAP. I suppose that has two forms: one, this baby is almost here, the miracle is almost complete, and two, this is freakin' weird. Get it out! Get it out!

What struck me about the whole process is that a woman's body and the baby just seem to know how to be born. It's actually quite a complicated series of twists and turns that ultimately grant your baby freedom, an escape only possible through a horrible maze that might face Indiana Jones in an ancient Aztec silver mine, yet everything just seems to happen instinctively. With modern technology and whizz-bang hospitals we have gotten so far away from nature that the quintessential act of nature—birth—seems odd. As I looked around the delivery room with all the strangers buzzing about I thought about the videos of home births I'd seen and couldn't help but think what a more peaceful experience that could be (assuming everything went well!).

The last piece of the puzzle is the shoulder. Once the baby wriggles its leading shoulder into position, your bachelor days really are in jeopardy. You've got a few seconds left. Despite repeated attempts, the 'denial button' no longer works. Even with the head and shoulder protruding you're still unaware of the baby's gender. The anticipation becomes almost unbearable and your mind races and your eyeballs start to sweat.

In one of the most surprising, miraculous, speedy, memorable moments of your life; you witness a little person emerge from the vagina of a big one. It seems stupid in the cold light of day to describe that, but it is a seriously unusual sight. In fact, I don't think I've seen anything like it before or since.

Once the vital head and shoulder combo was out the way I was shocked at the speed with which she almost literally shot out onto the hospital table, like a ping pong ball in a Bangkok bar.

As the baby exits her lungs are compressed, forcing out the liquid that was in there and thereby creating a vacuum. This vacuum forces the baby to take a big breath in, kickstarting the rhythm of life as we know it, a rhythm that I hope lasts for one hundred years or so. It's that same rhythm that you and I have been clinging to so far. It's a genuine miracle how it all just happens as it's supposed to.

I didn't expect her to be so purple . . . as purple as Jeff the Wiggle's skivvy. Purple, covered in a creamy white substance, blood and a surprising amount of hair—I'll say it: UGLY at first glance! You wouldn't be the first bloke to take the midwife aside and say, 'Hey, it's OK, you can tell me, what's the matter with him?' If it's a boy, he may have super gargantuan nuts (yes, you want him to have a penis like a baby arm holding an apple but nuts the size of ping pong balls at birth are something quite unexpected!). Then there's the head. When a baby is born its skull is soft so it can contort in the necessary shape to get out. If you ever wondered where the idea for the movie *Coneheads* came from, wonder no more. I'm reassured all the bits on him or her will settle down, as will the cone head, purple flesh, pink spots, white heads and yellow skin. Yep, there's no doubt that your bun fresh from the oven isn't pretty, but I guarantee it will be the most beautiful thing you've ever seen!

But here she was. The breathing gave way to a scream. I guess it's no wonder that babies cry: I'm sure it is a frightening journey that ends with light and noise and cold, but at least Mum and Dad are there and hopefully always will be. Then there's a big set of boobs to latch on to so they soon work out that life ex womb ain't all that bad!

Matilda let out her scream, and the entire weight of the world came off my shoulders. I mean all of it. In the closing scenes of *Being Dad* you can see me visibly rejoice, stumble and gush all over this moment. All of the worry was gone. The baby was here and fine and my wife was the MOST AMAZING person in the entire world. I'd have anointed her captain of the Australian cricket team, prime minister and world chancellor had those powers been available to me. Life had never been better and we, together, had completed one of the world's biggest transformations. Her journey was over nine months, mine in the preceding 60 seconds or so. I can guarantee you that all those worries and concerns we had during pregnancy were nowhere to be seen. A steely new resolve washed over me and I literally felt a new wave of pride and protector wash over me. In that instant I understood what it means to be a parent.

It's time to man up and admit to two things that I have previously denied. My mates are uninterested in most things I have to say, so I feel safe revealing personal secrets on page 208 of a book that they would have had to pay for and therefore be no chance of ever reading. This is as safe a place as any to reveal my weak moments. So here goes.

Firstly, with about an hour to go till the pushing started and Stacey asleep, I was overwhelmed with nerves and a racing mind as to what was in store. I think it is too easy to blame the tiredness, because I had a creeping worry that had been lurking in the back of my head for weeks. The whole process of birth seemed frighteningly uncontrolled. Anything could happen, and all I could do was watch.

I suppose my biggest, barely-thought-through fears were:

1. Stacey would die.
2. The baby would be die.

3. The baby would be born with some disability or severe abnormality.
4. There would be some horrifying panicky moment where the baby had the cord wrapped around its neck.

I'm not a religious person, but in the quiet few minutes in the darkened hospital delivery room, with my missus asleep and my baby on the wrong side of the 'great divide', I went downstairs to the hospital prayer room and prayed. Secret number 1. I prayed the clumsy prayer of a deathbed repenter and was really looking for the protection of my little family. If there is a supreme being, I'm sure my prayer would have been a fairly thinly veiled sales pitch: Hey, Creator of the Earth, I'm really sorry for all of the horrible things I've done, but I promise I'll be AWESOME from now on, TOTALLY DOUBLE PROMISE, if you can look after these guys for me. Deal? Please? Ace, thanks. Amen. I think as I threw the kitchen sink into the deal, I may have even talked about helping out charities . . . really got to get on to that.

I think, in hindsight, my (apparently very common) desperation reveals much about the first-time father. He has to do something. It's also interesting to note when it happened: I hit my most thoughtful and most desperate when all was completely serene. When there is nothing physical that can be done, the nervous male has to do something to help.

And I felt like I had done something. I certainly felt better and more centred. Whether it's a walk around the hospital garden or a brief moment in a prayer room, I seriously recommend a quiet moment to yourself if you can find one.

Something that helped me out as well was a visitors' book sitting in the prayer room. It held the ramblings and prayers of people who had done the exact same thing as me. Some were looking for help before a major operation, others for the speedy recovery of a loved one, others were blokes expecting the birth of their first baby. Reading the stories of bravery and courage in the visitors' book really helped me to centre myself.

My second oft-denied secret was that I cried. Shortly after the birth I moved just out of camera shot and lost it. To this day, I'm not sure why I reacted like that. Not everyone does and it's not right or wrong, but it happened to me and it happens to the vast majority of first-time dads. I'm not talking about your sweaty eyeball, mini sob and quick wipe with a Kleenex moment. I'm talking a flat-out blubbering, snotty-nosed, chest-heaving mess. It's the shock at being a dad, overwhelming relief that your wife and baby are safe, that you've made it through the day, and just a general emotional volcano. To be quite honest, I've become a more emotional person since that day. I want to cry when I see sick kids, can't bear ads for the RSPCA.

I don't think I've ever had as much respect for another person as I did for my wife at that moment. Even if I had the requisite equipment, I know that I could never have achieved what she did on that day. No matter what happens to us, our relationship or the future, I will not ever forget that: what she did or how she was on that day.

Despite all the pain, fear and uncertainty during birth, when the baby comes out it's as if your wife never felt a thing. I don't know whether it's adrenaline, relief of some other physiological occurrence, but holding her baby was like the world's greatest pain reliever.

Despite all that was going on and all that had happened, amazingly our baby started breastfeeding, everyone settled in and it became time to pass the news to the family and friends who had congregated outside. And there's not anything much more fun than that.

Baby is out and it's over . . . well, almost—here cometh the placenta.

Stage 3: Placenta and repair

You may have heard that back in the good ol' days nurses, midwives or obstetricians would whisk the baby away after the birth in order to check him/her out, clean up, weigh the baby and things like that. Totally not how it works now.

The first thing that happens is that the baby gets put on the mum's bare chest. The baby will stay there for as long as possible. Apparently, it's the best and most natural thing that could happen, which makes sense. It's amazing to watch how the baby just cuddles into mum and starts looking for the breast.

Turn the lights low, relax and revel in the moment. Get on board with some good old-fashioned skin on skin time. Whip your shirt off and jump into bed with your new family. Feel the baby on your bare chest and take in the earthy aromas of birth and a newborn baby. You'll never feel more of a man than you do right there.

If, for any reason, your obstetrician or midwife hurries you/ your partner/your baby up for weighing or cleaning make it clear, politely, that all of that can wait. This is important.

After the baby is born and resting comfortably on mum's belly or chest, it will be using the contact with your partner to help adjust to breathing outside of the womb, adjusting its temperature and looking around at the both of you.

After a few minutes, and almost off the radar, mum will start having contractions again as the placenta separates from the uterus. Her doctor or midwife will let her know when she should give one more push (usually not painful) and the placenta will come out. Even if you thought the baby wasn't all that pretty on arrival, take a look at the placenta. It makes your baby look like a supermodel! The placenta kept your baby alive for nine months, and as a parting gesture it shows you just how gorgeous your purple bundle of joy really is.

As much as you're proud of your new family, spare a thought for this ugly little chap. It looks like a frozen lump of minced meat wrapped in a red plastic bag (or a black pudding, if you've ever seen one of those). It did everything to nurture your baby and played a vital role in everything working out so well. Give it a knowing glance, tip your hat and bid it adieu. Placenta, we salute you. Some cultures eat the placenta, others bury it in their backyard for good luck. From all reports it's exceptionally healthy and chock full of nutrients, but then so is a multivitamin and a glass of water.

After the placenta is delivered you'll probably be invited to cut the umbilical cord. Most blokes have preconceived ideas about whether or not to cut the cord. Even if you don't think you will, you are a good chance to do so. It is a bit like cutting through a semi-defrosted, thin pork sausage.

NOTE: Troy omitted secret number three: in his exuberance to get through said defrosted snag he really went for it with the shears and not only made his way through the cord but also snipped into Matilda's thigh.

Finally, while you and mum are gazing in amazement at baby and each other, you won't even notice the doctor or midwife stitching up any incisions or tears and making sure mum is OK.

One bloke in the US *Being Dad* recalls his obstetrician calling him over to admire his handiwork, pointing to the nether regions of his wife, who was spreadeagled on the table . . . not bad, hey? Fortunately that was Texas, and presumably you are a long way from the Lone Star State.

The deal is done, now the hard work begins—welcome to parenthood, pal.

We remember watching a documentary on one of the Sydney to Hobart races in which the weather turned particularly nasty and claimed the life of several sailors and much of the fleet. At the end of the race one of the sailors who made it to the safety of the Hobart docks was interviewed, beer in hand. He described the four days at sea as the worst in his life, filled with terror and fear. He hadn't slept, was cold, tired and totally exhausted. He looked into the camera with tears in his eyes and said that this year would be his one and only Sydney to Hobart. Two hours later the same sailor had had a few more beers and enjoyed the comradeship of his fellow crew, reflected on the life-changing events of the past few days and announced that he'll be back next year. That perfectly sums up how you may feel after the birth of your first child!

Photocopy the following pages and take them into the delivery ward with you. You can refer to them during the birth; there's no shame in a cheat sheet!

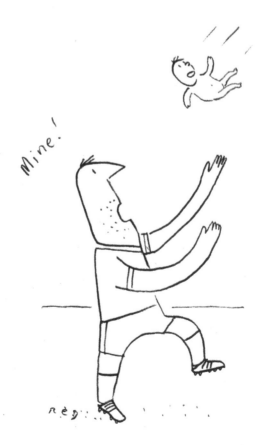

Things you must do during labour

1. Be actively involved; it's your baby, too.

2. Be patient. Labour can take many hours, so expect a long day/night. Keep the image of you holding your healthy baby in your mind. Just like a good golfer can see the shot he wants to hit, you can see what it's going to be like to hold your baby. The moment is drawing closer and closer.

3. Be flexible. Know your options and experiment to find what part of your birth plan may or may not work. Be prepared to try plan B. You may even be forced into a situation you weren't expecting. Keep your wits about you and you'll be fine. She'll be impressed if you recall some of the information from your childbirth class.

4. Toughen up. You may be trying to help, but given all the drama of the scenario she may get annoyed with you and tell you to shut up. Birth is a different world, but it only lasts for a day or so. She may need to vent and you may be the target. Don't take it personally. Take the feedback on board, do what she says and move on. It's no time to be mopey or confrontational.

5. Be her advocate but do not play doctor. Don't be afraid to ask questions of the medical staff or to make decisions or to tell them what you think.

6. Be there. That's the most important thing of all. Even if you're skittish about the birth, just being there is a massive help.

7. Encourage her physically and visually by staying close and looking at her lovingly, confidently and supportively (not with a look of fear on your face).

Some other things you can do to look useful and keep your brain from imploding

1. Offer her water after every contraction.

2. Offer her food—she needs to eat when she feels like it. You need to eat, too.

3. Help her change positions at least every 45 minutes (even during pushing, but more frequently then).

4. Get her to take a bath or a shower (or both). You'll both be surprised at how much it helps her feel better during contractions.

5. Give her a foot and hand massage.

6. Play music—whatever she wants. Really, even if you don't like it.

7. Offer her lip balm, brush her hair and put a cool cloth on her forehead.

8. Encourage her verbally and emotionally by saying positive things such as 'This is all normal', or 'You're doing great' or 'Let go'. Your words (and sometimes your silence) have the power to reassure her. Just like on the footy field, a wink, tap on the butt cheek or a knowing nod can convey much more than any words (especially when you've got a mouthguard in).

9. Ask questions of her medical providers, especially when interventions or medications are suggested.

10. Take pictures or record how her labour is going—she'll appreciate reading your version of the birth story (and so will your child!). We even talked ours into being in a film about it.

We've given you a complete list of things to do so you look and feel actively involved. But what about things you should and should not be saying? As was the case during pregnancy, it pays to think before you speak and it also helps to know what words will provide support and encouragement.

It may seem awkward to start saying some of these things, but once she's in labour you'll believe them! But remember, especially if you notice her moving into 'transition', sometimes saying nothing is what she needs. There are some simple things you can say that will help her; mums in labour are very receptive to positive feedback. Try to only be positive (and encourage everyone else to only say encouraging statements):

- 'You're doing great.'
- 'The baby is moving down. You're helping her come out.'
- 'The nurse says you're doing great.'
- 'I'm here with you—we're almost done.'
- 'I love you.'
- 'Everything is going to be OK.'
- 'Rest between contractions.'
- 'Keep breathing during contractions.'
- 'I'm sorry for doing this to you.' (Just kidding.)

Look into her eyes and just smile—seeing that you're calm and happy will comfort her.

So what now?

In a heartwarming and somewhat surprising spectacle, the baby has breastfed, goes to sleep and things momentarily resume some bizarre new sense of normality. The baby is wrapped up, put in a clear plastic cot and is completely zonked out. You could easily forget it is even there. Given the ups and downs of the last few hours, this reality creates itself quickly and you're relieved that it is here.

Even though you're clinging to coolness, the way in which your partner conducts herself in this period is worthy of a medal. If it were up to us blokes to have the babies there would be a team of experts taking care of everything else in our lives for the next few weeks. Time for a holiday. We hear the Maldives is nice this time of year.

Women seem driven to get things organised and move on. She may even be Superwoman. In fact, have you ever seen her and Superman in the same place at the same time. Coincidence?

She must be in pain, not to mention just as shocked as you, and has just pushed out a little person, but she powers on with some awareness of what to do and how to move to the next stage. The last thing that would be going through your mind would be packing up your stuff, but that's what happens. She gets tidied up, you help her; she packs her bags, you help her. You're honestly surprised she is doing anything, and you follow her like a lovesick puppy. You have no idea where you are, what she needs or what to do. But she does, so you follow.

With your stuff and your new baby and your eyes wide open trying to predict what happens next, you make your way through to the baby area of the hospital, get shown your new digs and start setting up your mini home for the next few days, unless you're heading home soon after the birth.

Your midwife takes this next walk with you, usually to a different floor. She's full of praise for the birth, and you nod and agree—this seems to be your new role in life. In the past 12, 24 or 48 hours she and her midwife mates (there may have been a few of them) have gone from total strangers to absolute, total freakin' legends and have become a vital part of your new life, and you're quietly hoping she will be with you for the next few years. Sorry, bro. No dice.

As the midwife hugs you and heads back for the next birth you're stunned to realise that she isn't coming home with you and she has another three babies to deliver before her shift is up (obviously yours will have been the most memorable of her career, with you getting three votes in the midwife equivalent of the Brownlow Medal). You may be faced with the option of a fold-out, roll-out bed on the floor if the hospital allows it, but your partner is more likely to suggest you go home, get some sleep and come back refreshed tomorrow. If the option's there, about 40 per cent of new dads stay and 60 per cent of new dads go.

What comes next is the most overwhelming fatigue you have ever experienced.

Chapter 9

In the hospital/your first week

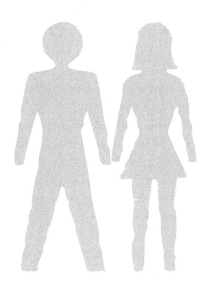

FOR H⚲R

Job done, baby delivered, what next? It's weird how you can go through nine months and the birth only to find yourselves in hospital feeling completely alone with no clue what to do next. It's a feeling of almost desperation, an anti-climax of sorts—a bit like the feeling you get the day after Christmas or the day you get home from holidays. Of course you're delighted with your new addition and just want to hold on to them the whole time, but the physical stress of the last few months really hits home now.

If you have had birth outside home you'll most likely spend a few days in hospital recovering and just getting used to your little one. There are the endless tests that get done, fussing of nursing staff and visits from paediatricians to check on junior. We can't fathom what it must be like for you, but we can tell you that your man will be pooped too. We hope he has managed to get a few days off work and can spend his days (and maybe a few nights if it's an option) in the hospital with you and the baby.

If you'd like him to stay, don't be afraid to ask or insist on him doing so. Spending time in the hospital and being very hands on is good for you, the baby and dad. It gives the baby an opportunity to bond with him, gives him the opportunity to build confidence and learn critical skills like bathing and nappy changing and gives you reassurance that he can be trusted to be left alone with the baby.

It can really help us guys to have expert nursing staff around to help teach us these new tricks. If your man hasn't had any experience with babies before, building confidence before leaving the hospital is very important. Much like teaching a new driver how to check the oil, water and tyre pressure in the car and change a flat tyre, your man shouldn't be given his licence to handle precious objects without passing a few standard, basic tests of competence. Hospital is the best place for this.

What else can he do while you're in hospital?

- Control the flow of visitors. Friends and family will be dying to visit and will all want to stay for hours, hold the baby and generally impart their own versions of parenting wisdom. You should try to use your time to rest, relax and recover. The baby will be around for the next 70 years, so there is no great rush to have hordes of people in the hospital with you. Get him to co-ordinate visitors and tell them when it's time to leave.

- Bring you real food. Hospital food doesn't seem to have improved over the years so treat yourself to takeaway from your favourite restaurant and your favourite coffee.

- Allow you to get some much-needed rest. Depending on how you gave birth and your recovery, you may need a few days in bed. He can take the baby out of the room and allow you to get some sleep during the day, especially if he isn't staying overnight. Don't feel guilty for sleeping when you feel like it or are able to. You need all the energy you can muster to recover and prepare for going home.

- Help with the nursing staff. Nursing staff are people, and sometimes you may not really like your nurse. They may get frustrated with you or just make you feel completely useless, and that can be really upsetting. If you strike someone who rubs you the wrong way, ask him to intervene and talk to them.

- Have him clean the house and stock the cupboards. If the baby came early and things were in disarray, ask him to have the house cleaned for your arrival. You also want plenty of food in the fridge and cupboards so you have everything you need. Coming home to a messy house that you may feel compelled to tidy isn't a great first day at home.

It may seem like he has the easy job when you send him off home after the first day. You're right, he does! But remember, it's not an easy thing to do leaving your new family behind and heading home to an empty house. Let's hope he'll go home and get a good night's sleep so he can come back the next day and do day duty while you rest up. There may, of course, be an obligatory head-wetting event at some point, and while it may seem like a frivolous excuse to get drunk it's a tradition that still has value for us menfolk. It's the only time in the whole process when he is the centre of attention and it's great for him to have his mates celebrate the success of his procreation.

In fact, all the hard work is really only just beginning. The first few weeks of being a parent are, without question, the most stressful ever for you and him. You may experience a bout of the baby blues or some postnatal depression, and it is also a particularly tricky time for new dads. He needs to be ready to really step up and provide as much support as possible to help make the adjustment back into home life. The next few weeks set the tone for the next few months and years, so you need to keep the lines of communication wide open. You must talk to him about how you're feeling, what he can do to help and when you're feeling down. Similarly, keep and eye and ear on him too. Postnatal depression can also strike men, so you both need to be conscious of each other's state of mind.

The next month or two is difficult and stressful but also blissful. In this chapter we will give him a heads up on what he can do to make life easier for you and the baby.

FOR H♠M

Once the birth is over, the baby has been cleaned, weighed and micro-chipped and the partner sewn back together, it's time to say goodbye to the delivery room and check into the new parents' wing of the hospital. In your few hours together you may have formed a very strong bond with the baby catchers. You're so indebted to them that you envisage them popping around for a lamb roast and a glass of red next Sunday night. Unfortunately, yours is just another birth, and after a hug and many thanks that's the last you'll see of them. One of the great things about birth doulas and some midwifery services is that they can also come around to visit post-birth to help out. We imagine there would be something very comforting in knowing they will be popping over to check on you once you get home.

If you did have a hospital birth you will be encouraged to attend classes about everything from breastfeeding to bathing to swaddling and sleep. Do the classes. Consume them with all your vigour. Take notes if you want to. Because soon enough— and honestly, sooner than you want them to—without as much as a multiple choice questionnaire testing your skills you'll be on your own and trying your hardest to remember what you were told in these classes.

The time in hospital is a great time to get proactive about being a dad. It is pretty easy to stand back and let all of it happen around you, and most blokes do that out of fear of doing something wrong or looking like an idiot or somehow hurting the baby. That's the wrong approach. Getting your baby-handling skills up to speed gives you confidence, and helps your baby feel comfortable around you and your partner feel comfortable leaving you around the baby. It's a rare win-win-win situation.

Volunteer to be the bloke who bathes his baby in front of the class. The nurses will lead you through it, and you will have had a practice. Try to change a nappy. After your baby has had a feed and a burp, wrap him up, pop him in his clear plastic bed/tub and go for a stroll around the hospital, leaving mum to have a shower, rest or just have few minutes to herself.

If you're nervous, just do a lap of your ward. If you're feeling braver catch the lift, wander down to the café and grab a coffee. You'll be rewarded by the smiles and nods of every passerby. Some older folks still marvel at seeing a new dad alone with a baby. The old boys look at you with dismay and the old girls give you a 'good on ya, sonny' look that will make you smile.

The ever-present fear is that the baby will wake up and start screaming, at which point you know you will go from Joe SuperCool sipping a latte to Mr Massive-bumbling-dickhead running for the lift in no time flat. Babies cry, that's their job. Stay calm, even though the first few times you're all alone with a crying baby it feels like an emergency worthy of a call to 000.

The key is to learn how long your baby sleeps for—if it's an hour, leave the room as soon as he falls asleep after a feed and give yourself 30 minutes. Keep an eye on your baby. If he starts to appear restless, smoothly and calmly stroll to the safety of your partner. The irony is, it's a race to see if you or your baby shits yourself first; it pays to remember that he's the one with the nappy on!

The truth is that your partner may well have just as little idea as you do when it comes to the baby unless she's done an apprenticeship with the super nanny, worked as an au pair, has a team's worth of brothers and/or sisters or is a nurse. Even then it seems that when it's your own baby the goal posts move, and no matter what your experience is you're stripped back to rank novice status.

Your partner will love you for having one-on-one baby time, and your horizons as a gutsy dad will start to grow. Such is the fickle nature of the post-baby period, though, that the baby may actually respond better to you than to mum when upset. While that's great for you—clearly you're a natural—it can make mum feel she's doing something wrong. Welcome to the at times impossible world of parenting!

If you're at a loose end during the hospital stay do the following every day:

- Get skin-on-skin with your baby.

- Sleep when the baby sleeps (which will be most of the time).

- See a lactation consultant. Breastfeeding is super important, but does not come naturally to the vast majority of women. Your partner may feel like a failure if it doesn't work for her. Keep a close eye on her, and insist on the support of external experts. They are effective, cheap and will improve your lives no end. Be gutsy here; it will improve your life.

- Practise nappy changes, bathing and swaddling/wrapping— these are essential skills you're going to need for a long, long time.

- You may hear differing opinions about how best to care for your baby or what position is best for breastfeeding, but you know yourselves and your baby—do what feels right to you. If things are not working, ask for help. This is easy to not do, but it's really important for you and your partner that you DO do it.

- If you and your partner had your baby in a hospital, make the most of bath and feeding times. Practice makes for a more relaxed dad, and mums say they find their partners more sexy when they watch them interacting tenderly with their children.

A good tip to save money during the hospital stay is to get a five- or seven-day parking pass. Without it, every time you go in and out of the hospital, which is likely to be very regularly, you pay through the snorkel. A weekly pass could save you hundreds of dollars.

Breastfeeding 101

Full tummies

Did you know that a newborn baby is full after no more than a teaspoon of milk? Newborn babies are not so affected by advertising as the rest of us: they know when to say when, and if you listen to them they will live long and prosper. It would seem the baby knows best.

In those first few weeks the baby does little more than wake up, eat, wee, poo and go back to sleep. They don't have any idea of manipulation. You can't cuddle your baby too much. Nine times out of ten, solving the crying issue is a pretty simple process of elimination. But if you feel that your baby is not eating well, or not eating enough, please contact a specialist. The specialists in our country are wonderful, caring, lovely people who are there to help.

We have heard from lots of blokes who agonised for weeks through a deteriorating situation over whether or not to contact the professionals for help on sleeping or feeding. Once they do, things improve almost immediately. Or they get divorced. One or the other.

Babies are busy drying out in the first few days, but they still receive a perfect personalised dose of nutrition from mum. Mum's boobs will not provide milk yet, but instead provide a substance called colostrum. It's yellowish, the texture of honey and full of nutrients that are perfect for your baby's first few days and antibodies that will protect him for the first month of life. Talk to a biologist; colostrum is as close to the perfect individualised energy source as is seen anywhere on the planet. So it's vital to do what you can to help with breastfeeding. As a dad one of your new duties is to promote the things that are best for everyone, and this one is cut and dried and fully sanctioned by the good folk at the World Health Organisation.

What if it just isn't working?

Sometimes, things don't work the way they should and it's no one's fault. It's highly likely that your partner will feel horrible about it, though—she will probably feel a failure as a mother. This is totally incorrect, of course, but it's one of the items on the post-baby brain malfunction checklist.

The female brain post-baby is like a laptop with a virus. You know things aren't working quite right, but you can't put your finger on the problem. It's just not the same old laptop. We'll explore the baby blues and postnatal depression later, but it's no surprise that the huge doses of hormones over the last nine months and the physical release post-birth can lead to a hard drive that may take some time to reboot and clean out. Expect it, so look for the signs and be sympathetic.

It's very likely that your partner, and maybe even you, will have an occasional bout of self-doubt and feel you're doing something or everything wrong. Breastfeeding is an area of particular sensitivity.

If it isn't working, and the specialists have had their say and it still isn't working, that's all you can do. No one needs to feel like a criminal; everyone is trying their best. Ultimately, you have to do what you and your partner feel is best.

Mother and baby have a very close connection. They share a very special communication that we like to call 'boob-tooth', and breast milk is the best source of the essential nutrients your baby needs. If your partner doesn't plan to breastfeed, ask why. If it simply can't be done, for whatever reasons, consider at least getting the first few days of colostrum into the baby using a cup or spoon (try not to introduce a bottle in the first week).

The cycle of feeding and sleeping, when it's not working, can turn into a hellish slippery slope, and if it is not resolved it can deteriorate into a scary downward spiral. Watch it carefully, and don't feel frightened to put out an SOS to an expert. You're not alone; this has happened thousands of times before and it will be OK. Just don't let anything get out of hand.

It's important to remember, though, that your partner might not realise she needs help. This is a pretty thin line to walk, but if things aren't going well and she's taking it personally—and wanting to sort it out without 'embarrassing herself'—you may need to go get the help yourself.

Our only advice is not to make the decision to give up on breastfeeding at night. During the night, with sleep deprivation (and everything else!) at its most scary, everything seems worse. Your encouragement of your partner is vital. If the two of you can make it till daylight, think about it in the cold hard light of day and you will most likely make a better decision—whatever that decision might be.

Again, this is a time where everyone has an opinion. Family, friends, passersby will all have their say. As frustrating as it can be, the best approach is to nod and smile and move on. If you find one specialist you like, stick with them.

Being a good dad is not simply about agreeing with your partner—it's about owning your new life. It means checking into things, taking an active interest in the best ways to do things and having an opinion and respecting your partner and her wishes. Be careful, considerate and sensitive, but always aim for what is best for everyone.

What's in breast milk?

As a fabulous part of boob-tooth technology, to support the baby's drying-out phase actual breast milk 'comes in' usually on day four or five and changes daily to match your baby's body and brain needs. It contains the perfect balance of water, fat, protein, carbohydrates, hormones, vitamins and minerals. If you want a well-balanced, healthy nipper, the best head start you can give them is by connecting nipples and mouths: her nipples to baby's mouth, just to be clear.

For you fellas out there who put on a few extra kilos during the pregnancy, your baby may mistake your nipples for hers. Embarrassing, yes, but also hilarious (for everyone except you).

Baby formula has about 50 ingredients. Breast milk has over 350! It's really unbelievable if you think about it: there are people living on an international space station right now but we can't reproduce breast milk.

Why men think breastfeeding is great

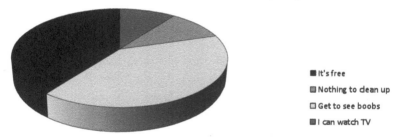

- It's free
- Nothing to clean up
- Get to see boobs
- I can watch TV

The real reason why it's great!

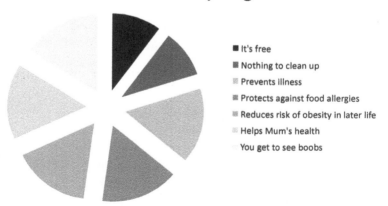

- It's free
- Nothing to clean up
- Prevents illness
- Protects against food allergies
- Reduces risk of obesity in later life
- Helps Mum's health
- You get to see boobs

As you can see in the above pie charts there are some legitimate reasons for encouraging breastfeeding other than bigger boobs and being able to watch the football. And don't forget that you too can feed the baby with breast milk. Get involved: if your partner pumps her milk with a breast pump, then you can feed your baby with a bottle. It is a great way to give mum some extra sleep, for you to bond with your baby and to get some one-on-one time together.

TROY: I was lucky enough to have both of my babies born proximate to the Ashes series in England. Now, admittedly, neither tour ended well, but it gave me the reason to get up and do the midnight and 4 am feeding. HUGE brownie points, and all that's required is to get:

- A breast pump from your local pharmacy (rental is available at some). Expressing milk at 4 am, my missus was looking for the fastest, easiest way to get the milk into the bottle, so the industrial version was great.
- The bottles, nibs and other bits and pieces.
- A good steriliser. Somehow or other, this stuff when used properly totally sterilises the bottles, nibs etc.
- A bottle warmer. Don't microwave your bottles. You can get some super baby-friendly bottle warmers that don't mess with the delicate composition of the milk.

If you can do this for a few weeks, you're doing two things. One, creating a lifelong bond between you and your baby. Two, allowing your wife to get some sleep. Rather than four-hour breaks, by taking one session you give her an eight-hour break. That is gold. You might even be able to trade that for something. Use your imagination, but a rested wife is a happy wife is a happy bloke and happy parents make happy kids . . . don't confuse that with happy parents make kids . . . that's what got you here at 4 am in the first place. On that, you should be aware that the period following childbirth can be particularly fertile for her, so unless you're looking for another quick wicket before stumps it may pay to invest in some rubbery devices.

When you become a parent it somehow triggers the entrepreneur in you. You constantly find things that could be done better, or a totally new product that will revolutionise the entire baby caper. Just look at what we've come up with in this book alone. A vaginal air pressure wristwatch, a sexometer and a few new theories to complement those drummed up by Newton, Einstein et al.

Well here's another one. If only there was some kind of meter on the boob that allowed us all to get some idea of how much milk was being ingested, something like a petrol gauge that measures how full the boobs are or when the baby's tank is full. Surely if there is an iPhone app that can listen to the radio and tell us what song is playing we must be able to point our iPhones at our wives' lactating breasts to know how many millilitres our nippers are taking on board? Someone in China needs to get on to it ASAP.

In the absence of an iPhone app we'll have to go old school and look for physical signs that your baby is getting enough milk. Unfortunately, this involves trawling through dirty nappies and other antiquated, non-technological activities. The following list is useful, but does not make for particularly lovely images:

- Your baby is waking on its own and eager to nurse.

- Your baby is peeing clear or very pale urine at least once on day one, twice on day two, three times on day three and six times from day four.

- The nappies feel really heavy and you know they are wet.

- Your baby is pooing every day (at least half a cup, yuck . . . but important to know) and the poos are yellow and seedy (also yuck) by the fourth day of life or within 24 hours of mum's milk 'coming in'.

- Your baby's eyes are alert, bright and white.
- Your baby's skin is a healthy colour.
- Your baby moves its arms and legs actively.
- Newborn babies sleep a lot, but when your baby is awake it is alert and content.
- Baby is back to birth weight by somewhere in days two to seven and gains weight from there.

The reason the baby loses weight is because essentially it is drying out. Especially if the above signs are all there it's totally normal, so don't worry about it. As to what life has become now that you're measuring poo by the cup and not in inches or kilos, well, that's a whole other story . . . welcome to being a dad!!

Poo and wee

Over the next few years you will be encountering and discussing poo, wee and vomit more than you'd probably care to. Changing nappies really isn't as bad as it's made out to be. Once your baby gets on the solids you'll start to encounter richer, fruitier and more stomach-turning aromas, but just like your own rotten stench it's somehow palatable as it's emanating from the fruits of your loins.

The first few wees your baby does may contain traces of blood. This is normal, and nothing to freak out about. The first poo can best be described as the aftermath you could expect from a fully laden tar truck hitting a brick wall at 100 km/h. It's as black as the black hole and stickier than any substance known to mankind. Faced with this poo, known as meconium, one might reasonably expect that the little one has some serious internal issues but, no, it's normal.

Here are a few poo and wee tips for the uninitiated:

- Poo and cotton don't mix—always remove socks before changing a nappy.

- Poo can and will escape a nappy.

- A Huggies nappy can hold around 300 millilitres of wee—that's almost a full Coke can! When shopping, green nappies are for newborns, blue is for boys and pink is for girls. On the nappy itself, the cartoon character goes at the front.

- When you take off a baby boy's nappy, chances are he will start peeing. ALWAYS keep the nappy over him until you have the new one ready to go.

- A change table with everything you require in close proximity is very helpful. Speed saves a mess. Nappy off, wipe down, apply cream if necessary, nappy on. It's like a pit stop in the Grand Prix—time really matters!

Chapter 10
The first few months at home

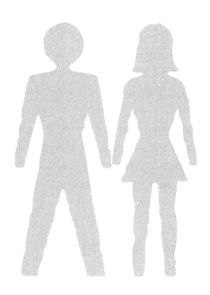

FOR H♀R

Seriously, this is where the work starts. Only a few of us, maybe five or six men in the history of mankind, actually managed to visualise coming home with a baby. It's a shock to find yourself back at home after the tumultuous events of the birth and with another little person in tow, and the reaction of most blokes once they close the front door for the first time is, 'Shit, what do we do now?'

Again, it's a testament to our mastery of the art of denial. Despite assisting in setting up elements of the baby's room—building the cot, painting the room, putting together the change table—chances are he has never really thought through what life will look like with a baby in the house.

Most blokes have no problem dreaming up 21st speeches and planning trips to play golf with their adult kids (21 years into the future), but mention the phrase 'Bringing the baby home' and you'll be met with a blank stare.

He may be cool, calm, collected and brave at the hospital, but with the first whiff of fresh air as he steps onto the pavement out the front of the hospital his confidence ebbs away, reaching a historic low as he attempts to put the baby into the car seat and contemplates the road, figuratively and literally, ahead.

How to get him thinking about getting the baby home

Unless he's a real handyman, don't let him install the car seat himself. In fact, even if he works for a baby car seat company don't let him install the car seat. They don't let doctors operate on themselves or family members for a very good reason! At most Australian hospitals you can get a baby seat guru to install the seat for you. If possible, have this genius install it a week or two in advance so your man can get used to driving with a baby seat in the car: it's a sure anti-denial tool. Driving around the suburbs with a baby seat and doll in the back sounds insane, but it works!

You know the scene in a horror film where the star gets into his or her car and everyone in the theatre, except said star, knows that some hottie with a big set of fangs is lurking in the back seat ready to suck their blood. Cue dramatic music and look of panic and terror when the star realises death is imminent—that's what it's like as a man the first time you look in your rear-view mirror and see a baby seat (with or without a baby).

Another handy way to prepare him for home is to run a few fire drills in the middle of the night. Think we're kidding? Get yourself a recording of a baby crying and in the weeks leading up to the birth let it rip at 11 out of 10 volume on your home sound system. We're talking 4 am, when he's deep in REM sleep. For extra fun, hide the remote so he needs to find it to turn the sound down . . .

What to do with them both once you get home

What can you expect from your man once you finally get home, assuming you left home in the first place to have the baby?

He'll think he's doing more than ever; you'll feel he's not doing enough

There has been plenty of research done into modern relationships and it seems that the share of household duties performed is still far from equitable. Let's assume that before the baby comes home your man does 40 per cent of household chores (sure, we're being generous). Now, let's assume when you get home with the baby he ups his output by 50 per cent, meaning he now does 60 per cent of the chores around the house. He feels that he's putting in BIG TIME. What he doesn't factor in is that there are 100 per cent more chores now, meaning he's really only doing 30 per cent of the total chores, which is 10 per cent less than he was doing pre-baby.

We're no geniuses at maths but let's look at that: pre-baby he's doing 40 per cent, post-baby he's doing 30 per cent. Assuming the average weekly chores are ten hours before baby, when the baby arrives he's doing four hours of chores a week and you're doing six, and post-baby he's doing six hours and you're doing 14!!

When you factor in the fact that you have the baby and have less time than ever to do anything, you can see how issues arise. He's baffled because he's doubled the amount of time he's putting in pretending to clean the house, and you're filthy with him because you're spending more time than ever when you have less than ever available!

It's so confusing we can barely keep up with it, let alone explain it. The only way you can combat this mathematical conundrum is to create a spreadsheet that lists the daily and weekly chores and the estimated time to complete them. Divide them up into proportions that seem fair and stick to it. Don't forget that chores include things outside the house that he may do regularly, such as mowing the lawn or maintaining his golf handicap. Oh, hang on . . .

He assumes you know more than he does about your baby

This is true for every man alive. Our instincts tell us that we know nothing and you know everything, but you're probably just as scared, unsure and nervous about being a parent as he is. This phenomenon really becomes evident when the baby gets ill. He'll have no idea what to do or who to call but will believe you know exactly what to do. He at least has the 'She'll be right' philosophy to keep him somewhat calm, whereas you have the 'Worry about everything' gene that will be sending you into a tailspin.

We can only assume this puts even more pressure on you girls. So what's the action plan? Talk about how confident you are or are not. Don't try to be all knowing if you don't have a clue. It's OK, no one except you two expects you two to be experts, and letting him know that you're in the brown stuff together will probably make him feel better about himself.

He's an easy target

Picture this: it's 3 am, you haven't slept at all tonight and have averaged only a few hours a night for the last week. The baby won't settle and he strolls around wondering what's wrong and why won't the bloody baby just go to sleep. He may as well be a deer with a red target on its chest walking down the main street of Alaska in hunting season. You're going to unload everything you have on to him. Why? Because you can, and because he's the only deer stupid enough to walk down your main street in hunting season wearing a red target.

The truth is that in the first few months you're both the deer and it's always hunting season. You will scream and rant and rave at one another at some point. There's not much point taking it out on the baby, but it sure feels good to tell him what a lazy no-good prick he really is! Yeah!

What's the solution? Sleep, but you aren't going to get it right away. Before the baby comes, have a chat about how to handle those situations. It won't help at the time but if you have at least acknowledged that it's going to happen, you'll have something to fall back on (and argue about) when it does. Bring on daybreak, when sanity always seems to return!

Sex? No thanks

We've talked a lot about sex in this book already and now you're entering phase three of the sexual challenge of parenting. There's conception, pregnancy and now post-baby sex. Which is the most tricky? As with everything in parenting, who the hell knows?

Problems that you may encounter include:

- You being ready to get back on board but he's still suffering from post-traumatic stress or shell shock from the delivery.
- He's itching to get back into it but you'd rather be sewn shut for all eternity.

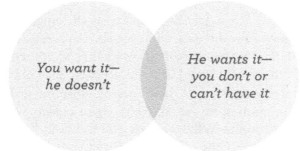

This is a classic Venn diagram that describes the conundrum. See the dark bit in the middle? It doesn't exist. No, that's not true. If you're on the right-hand side of this diagram, ask yourself what can be done to move into the middle. If it's not a physical thing (that is, you can't), what can he do to shift? Give you more time to exercise or sleep? Help out more around the house? Stop wearing your G-strings? Maybe you just aren't ready, in which case just reassure him that you love him and that you'll be ready soon. As we said about sex during pregnancy, you don't need to restrict yourselves to penetrative sex; there's a lot of fun to be had just fooling around!

If he's on the left-hand side, what can you do to lure him back towards the middle? Time alone, his favourite lingerie, a massage or just helping yourself to yourself in front of him . . . You know him better than we do, but he's a bloke so he can be drawn back to the middle without too much difficulty if you really apply yourself.

Don't let things slip for too long; they can be hard to recover.

He's not bonding with the baby

It's a well-known fact that it takes most guys longer than their women to really feel bonded with the baby. Maybe that's just because no one ever taught us what to do to help the process along. The key is to appeal to our fixing and curious nature. We'll show him how to spot signs of development and how to help the baby learn and develop. Your job is to make sure he gets enough one-on-one time and the space to make his own blunders.

He feels left out

This is a big one. When you get home, you will probably be focusing 100 per cent on the baby. That's all the time and affection he's used to getting. He may feel ignored, useless or unwanted.

Loads of guys have told us that they really struggled with the change in the relationship dynamics. It may well be one of the things that can lead to postnatal depression in men, a phenomenon that is now being recognised by the health care community.

You feel down and he doesn't get it

The baby blues and postnatal depression are a bit like morning sickness: a complete mystery to most men. Not only may he not recognise the signs that you're struggling, he may seem unsympathetic towards them. Do you have a history of PND in the family? If you do, you're at increased risk of experiencing it.

Postnatal depression is not something that you can stop happening, but it can be effectively treated. Put it on your checklist of things to discuss before birth and agree on how to tackle it if the signs don't go away after a few days.

*   *   *

All the above sounds miserable, but of course you may never experience any of it. You may be one of the lucky couples that just breezes through. Either way, by understanding each other and the possible pitfalls you'll be better prepared to cope with them.

To work or not to work—that is now the question

Most of you will have a timetable for one or both of you returning to work. As that time approaches it can become particularly stressful. You may not want to return to work as planned, and the thought of leaving your baby for eight hours a day in the care of someone else may be unbearable. What to do? The answer to that lies with your financial situation and the plans you've made, but try to remember that most guys are thrust straight back into work and so have to wave goodbye to their new family every morning. We're not suggesting that it's as hard for men as it is for women, just that it's a point worth bearing in mind.

Most parents also battle with the division of labour. Of the hundreds of dads we've interviewed, a very high percentage agree that it's a good idea for dads to spend a week or two alone at home with the baby to gain an understanding of just how difficult being a full-time parent can be. Without that experience many guys will think that the stay-at-home mum has it pretty easy and will fail to understand why the house isn't spotless or dinner hasn't been prepared.

Staying at home and looking after a baby is bloody hard work. It's very common for issues to arise around who works, who stays at home and who has it harder. Unfortunately, there are no formulas or checklists you can use to work out what is best for your situation; it's all a matter of your individual circumstances.

The best advice that our dads gave is to not assume that one of you has it easier or better. Understand the pluses and minuses of both situations and try to be respectful of each other's roles. Constantly reassess the division of labour and try to find a happy medium where neither party feels they are bearing too heavy a burden.

The above may all seem like common sense, and it is, but when you're tired, stressed and trying to cope with a new baby and a new relationship common sense can be hard to find. God speed!

FOR HÏM

Let's be honest: it's tough enough imagining that a little person is about to come out of your partner. We can almost guarantee that, like most of us, your thought process has gone no further than the birth. Can you honestly imagine walking out of the hospital, strapping your baby into a car seat, driving home and closing the front door with a new member of the family? Go on, just try to imagine it.

Regardless of how cool and composed you were in the hospital, walking out the front door is intimidating. Strapping him into his car seat for the first time is frightening, the drive home is terrifying and closing the front door behind you that first time will be petrifying.

Getting the baby home and surviving the first few months is something neither of you is likely to have given much thought to. All your focus has been on pregnancy and birth; anything past that is difficult to grasp. This is a period of adjustment for all new dads. It's back to reality, back to work and time to start dealing with a whole new world. It can be an assault on your sanity, your patience and your relationship so it pays to be aware of the issues that usually arise.

The drive home

If you get your car over 50 km/h you're doing better than most. Just about every dad will agree that the drive home from the hospital is terrifying. For starters, you can almost guarantee that your partner will be in the back seat with the baby, barking orders at you to slow down even though you're being passed by invalid pensioners in electric wheelchairs. Every bump, every turn you'll be praying doesn't upset the little one and you'll feel as if every kilometre is ten. The relief of pulling into your driveway or garage in one piece is palpable. You now understand why some cars have a 'Baby on Board' sticker.

As you move towards that first step into your home it will start to dawn on you that you have absolutely no idea what to do when you get inside. The average Aussie bloke spends more than 15 minutes unpacking the car when he gets back, presumably because he knows what he is doing: unpacking the car. It keeps the mind busy for a while as the final strands of denial dangle tenuously, hanging on for dear life. And you'll most likely do it bit by bit, package by package, hoping that your partner will, in the meantime, have worked out what you're supposed to do next.

Unfortunately, the last of your individually couriered packages will lead you to your partner, who is holding your baby and has a similar look on her face that says, 'RIGHTO . . . What the hell do we do now?'

Babies fresh from the hospital don't usually juggle, play computer games, make jokes or even talk much, so there is no avoiding the 'What do we do now?' moment in the kitchen or living room. You've just taken off in the marathon of parenting, and it's not action stations all the time.

New babies are exhausted and generally sleep for much of the first few weeks. The key is to make the most of the time when the baby sleeps. Although you aren't exhausted yet, you do have exhausting times ahead, believe us, so rest whenever you get the chance. Don't worry about keeping the house super tidy for the first week or so. Sleep when you can.

It doesn't matter what you do, the first few days at home will soon become a total blur. It's amazing the way something that only weighs 3 or 4 kilograms and basically sleeps all the time can turn the world upside down. There are two of you, combined (most likely) with over 50 years of life experience, and one two-week-old baby and every day it seems as if not much changes, but when you look at the photos of your three-day-old baby in a month's time you won't believe how much he has grown and the things that are starting to happen.

An important bit of advice given to us was to not look too far ahead. Don't look forward to when the baby smiles or sits or walks or talks . . . that will happen soon enough. Enjoy this wonderful little bloke or girl every minute you can. Take the photos and the videos—maybe even make a diary of what happens when. We guarantee that if you do that, your grown up boy or girl would love to read it sometime down the track.

But here's some practical advice for working through that first month.

How much sleep can you expect?

The average newborn sleeps 16 hours per day, but only in periods of two to four hours. As a result, most new parents feel sleep deprived because it's difficult to get much value from an interrupted sleep. If you're worried about your baby's sleeping patterns or you'd like to learn more about encouraging your baby to sleep longer we suggest the following resources:

- *The Baby Sleep Book* by William Sears.
- *Sleeping with Your Baby: A Parent's Guide to Co-Sleeping* by James McKenna.

- Tresillian offers an in-house and out-of-house sleeping course.

If your baby isn't a sleeper, night-time can be stressful. When the baby is crying uncontrollably at 3 am and everyone else you know is sleeping soundly and you're dead tired, things can feel pretty grim. Sometimes you literally just have to tough it out till daybreak. As the sun rises things feel normal again and you will feel a renewed sense of control. It's important to ensure that you're both getting at least some sleep. Don't think you can sleep all night and then head to work, leaving an exhausted partner and baby to try to battle through the day. That's a recipe for disaster. Most workplaces are sympathetic to new parents and understand that life at home can be a bit crazy for a while—take advantage of that.

If you feel you might need help, don't feel embarrassed or ashamed to ask for it. It can be bloody hard work and stressful. When you ask your mates they'll all say, 'Oh, little Jimmy was a real sleeper' but it's all bullshit. Just like the birth when your partner forgot lots of the pain once the baby arrived, most parents soon forget the fatigue and terror of the first few weeks once they get into the groove. You're not alone; we've all been there and it isn't easy.

Don't be surprised if you find yourself in your PJs walking around the neighbourhood at 3 am with the baby in the pram feeling only anxiety and doubt. Don't think that everyone else seems to be handling it better. They aren't.

It's also worth considering that some people have the parenting gene and others don't. We don't know if the boffins at Genetics HQ in Switzerland have identified the actual gene but we're certain it's the case. Parenting seems harder for some than others, but ultimately the ability is there within us all. If you listen to your intuition, it will come.

Six tips for getting some extra kip

1. Just like being prepared for extra traffic around sporting events, be prepared for broken sleep. It might help you to think of it as sleep interruption, not sleep deprivation, since you really should be sleeping when the baby sleeps (as much as possible!).

2. Share the burden and take turns getting up to settle the baby. If your baby is waking up every three hours and you share the job you can each get six hours sleep straight, which is not a bad start.

3. Change your sleeping patterns—have earlier nights and nap when you get the chance. Especially early in the baby experience, get your TiVO or Foxtel IQ to earn its keep and get to bed early.

4. Keep baby close by for easy access—if you hear your baby starting to wake up you can feed him or her before the crying starts.

5. Sleep together, at least in the same room. Sleeping apart can create problems. You need to be a team and share the night-time duties where possible. Even if your partner is willing and able to get up to tend to the baby every time during the night, just being there and giving her some comfort and love as she gets up and down is beneficial.

6. If people ask you what gifts they can get you, ask the good cooks for prepared meals, frozen so you can heat them up at dinner time. Ask the maternal ones for some baby-sitting time so you can rest or just spend some time together. Let's face it: how many Bob the Builder trucks or pieces of plastic Mattel crap do you think you're going to need?

Above all, do everything you can to avoid sleep deprivation, especially for mum—it can have serious consequences and is one of the major causes of postnatal depression. Allow friends and relatives to come over and help you so you can get more sleep. And encouragement, gifts and extra effort from you with household chores such as laundry and cooking really do help.

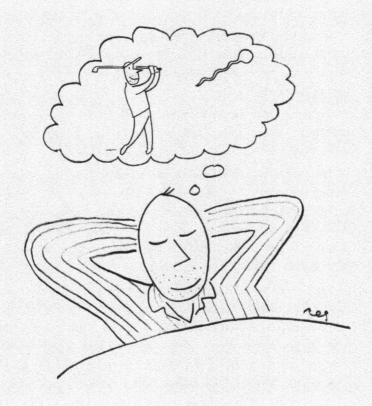

It's really easy to shirk the issue and carry on with your life as it was. That's a huge mistake, and you'll miss out on a lot of the experience. Other than not having boobs you can do everything that she does, and by lifting some of the overall load you'll be doing your bit for your new family.

Night feeding: it's your chance for one-on-one and to catch up on sport on Foxtel

Make sure you time it so that the bottle is warmed before your baby really gets wound up. Otherwise:

- you will wake up your partner; and
- it will make it harder for you to put the baby back to sleep. Get yourself a bottle warmer.

Beware: milk takes a while to heat up, but it takes an AGE to cool down. Getting the milk temperature correct is a real skill, worthy of a Boy Scout badge at the very least.

Remember that breast milk is like liquid gold. It's hard work for your partner to produce, express and store, so any spillage or wastage can result in trouble. Many a man has nearly lost the use of appendage for wasting stored breast milk. As a dad once told us, sometimes being a good dad is not so hard; being a good husband is the tough part.

Getting feeding right may take a night or two, but once you work out each other's schedules you and your baby will get along famously. It really is a very satisfying feeling looking into your baby's eyes as he or she slurps on a bottle, watching their eyes roll back into their head as the warm breast milk hits their miniature stomach and starts putting them into blissland. It really is like watching someone get drunk . . . little giggles, sighs of contentment, drooping of the eyelids, rolling of the eyes, burping, farting and sleep. Once you've burped the baby and put it back into the cot you'll feel like a bona fide dad.

Everyone is a f+cking expert

The absolute worst part of being a parent is learning that everyone else in the world is an expert. What happens to people when they have kids that makes them take such a radical stance on issues such as feeding, crying, sleeping, day care, bathing?

You and your partner are living your life, and your circumstances and beliefs are unique. You need to work out what works for you and what doesn't. There is no right and wrong way, there's only what works for you. Sure, you'll make mistakes and do things a certain way that in hindsight you may wish you hadn't, but that's life and that's parenting.

Everyone you encounter will want to give you hints, tips, suggestions, advice and the occasional admonishment or death stare. Unless you have actively sought said advice, smile, ignore and move on.

Daddy Ninja skills

In our opinion, the biggest challenge of all 'She'll be right' daddying is sleep. Many will talk of routine, bath gels, music—and we agree with them all.

But in the early days the Daddy Ninja skills are vital. They basically involve transitioning the baby that is sleeping on your shoulder into the baby that is sleeping peacefully in their cot. The beautiful little buggers must have some kind of compass/altimeter in them.

The baby could be TOTALLY zonked out on your shoulder . . . we mean dribbling, snoring, asleep, but anything other than carefully honed and refined Baby ninja techniques will instantly wake them up. The worst part is if they don't realise they've been asleep for only five minutes. They may think they have been asleep for hours and assume they are ready to party. Then you have a real problem so the Daddy Ninja moves are vital.

Here ar the official *Being Dad* Daddy Ninja tips:

1. Have a routine and stick to it.

2. Change the baby's nappy before the baby is asleep.

3. Wrap the baby well.

4. Prepare the cot so that you can put the baby directly under the blankets without much fuss. (ALWAYS put the baby at the bottom of the cot, devoid of toys and excess blankets and gear. Never ever smoke anywhere near a baby, and have the room dark and comfortably warm.)

5. Over time, you will discover what puts your baby to sleep. For some, it is walking around with the baby's head resting on the front of the shoulder. Walking laps of the living room, bouncing a little bit and patting him on the back can be a sure-fire method.

6. Once you're SURE that the baby is asleep, continue your walking/bouncing/patting for another two minutes. These two minutes are a very strong investment. If you go too early in order to save these two minutes, you may find yourself up for another hour getting the little one back to sleep. If you're feeling strong try five minutes, or maybe set a target of laps around the room. It helps us to think of the new dads all around the country doing the same thing at the same time. Bless you blokes.

7. Once you're confident that you have a zonked baby, sneak into the bedroom and move towards the edge of the cot.

8. Halfway into the action of tilting your body into position to lower the baby, stop. For us, this is when you're angled at 45 degrees. This is to acclimatise the internal baby altimeter to a new angle. Hold it there for ten seconds. You may feel him wriggle a bit, so stay at that angle and wait for him to settle.

9. Transition him off your shoulder with your hand supporting his head. At this point he is horizontal, levitating above his cot. A bit like the world's strongest man holding a massive lump of cheese, linger here for ten seconds or so.

10. Gently lower the little one, and with as little drag on the sheets as possible slide him under the blanket. Always lie babies on their back.

11. He is now in bed, but you will still have one hand under his head and one around and underneath his back. The job is nowhere near complete. In terms of time you're almost finished, but in terms of vital remaining steps this is the big Daddy Ninja challenge. You need to transition your hands from under him to grasping (firmly but gently) both of his shoulders. We can hear you say 'impossible', but

it can be done. The key is to do one hand at a time. We go for the 'under the back' hand first, relocating it to his shoulder. The hand on the shoulder reassures him that nothing drastic has changed.

12. Slide your second hand from under his head, extremely gently, to the other shoulder.

13. Pause with both hands on his shoulders for a moment. He may wriggle, but your hands should help him chill.

14. Remove both hands.

15. Gently back away from the cot.

16. Time your strides with passing traffic to minimise noise.

17. If you choose to shut the door, recite the Daddy Ninja mantra: a door is never closed until you remove your hand from the handle. The door closing will trip up many a newbie. Gently pull the door closed. Many presume at this point that their job is complete and let the handle go, creating a bang that wakes the baby. Always let the handle return to its original position before letting go.

18. Walk off and punch the air and celebrate (silently) like a moron.

You are Daddy Ninja. Welcome to the brotherhood. These skills need to develop and adapt as the baby gets older, but the core skills remain the same.

Why doing more isn't necessarily enough

One of the biggest mistakes we men make is feeling we are doing more than we were before the baby arrived. Yes, you may be picking up your own undies, cooking a meal or bathing your baby, but that doesn't constitute 50 per cent of the new tasks that need to be done. Sit down together and write a list of all the things that need to be done every day and work out how you can do more.

Once a baby arrives the household chores double. Assuming you currently do 40 per cent of them, in order for your partner to spend the same amount of time on them that she did before the baby your output needs to more than triple! If you don't believe us, do the math. It's frightening!

Here are a few things you can do to help out more:

- Cook for her. She's breastfeeding, so healthy meals will benefit her and the baby. While he's still using boob-tooth it's just like being in the womb, so cooking for her is really cooking for the whole family.

- Make sure the fridge and cupboards are well stocked with healthy food, milk, water and other necessities (and a few treats).

- Sign up for a mail-order movie service or on-demand movies with your pay TV, or just pick up some DVDs or books on your way home.

- Be there: no sneaking off with the guys after work unless you can trade it for the late-night feeds, for example. However, if you can work a night out with the boys into the schedule, you will get less than zero sympathy for your hangover the next morning. Especially if the late-night feeds are part of the deal, it could be a rough choice that may not be worth the pain. Oh, who are we kidding? If you've earned it, enjoy yourself. Just remember, changing nappies and a crying baby on a hangover are a genuine nightmare.

- Try to work reasonable hours to help out with feeding and bathing.
- If she's pumping breast milk, do at least one bottle feed a day.
- Get up at least once during the night to feed and soothe the baby.
- Let her sleep in on the weekends.
- Tell her she's doing a great job and that you love her . . . every day!!
- Massage her feet while she's holding or feeding the baby.

The baby blues—what are they and what can you do?

The baby blues are common mood swings experienced by mums after childbirth. Symptoms usually appear three to four days after the delivery and can last for several days. The baby blues and postnatal depression are very difficult for us to comprehend. Postnatal depression also affects men, so if you find yourself feeling a bit down don't be too surprised.

Symptoms of the baby blues may include:

- Mood swings—joy to tears in an instant. Often there will be at least one day where your partner will be particularly teary. The fixer in you will look for a solution, but there isn't one. Give her a hug, tell her she's doing a great job, give her some extra time out and do your very best to be understanding.
- Feeling a little depressed.
- Lack of concentration.
- Loss of appetite.
- Inability to sleep.

Keep an eye out for these symptoms and be as supportive as possible. Remember, your partner's body has been through a tough nine months and hormones are rampant. These symptoms should disappear within ten days; if not, you need to be aware of postpartum or postnatal depression. The signs may not always be obvious. Be on the lookout, and remember that most new mums will experience at least one of the symptoms.

Postpartum depression: what is it and what are the warning signs?

Postpartum (or postnatal) depression (PND) can affect men as well as women, so it's important that you're aware of the warning signs and symptoms. It can be treated with therapy and support. PND can be frightening, so seek help if you're concerned at all. As with the baby blues, it can be very hard as a bloke to understand PND and we tend to feel completely helpless in terms of knowing how to help. The signs to watch for are:

- feeling sad and low or unnatural highs
- frequent crying and tearfulness
- feelings of restlessness, anxiety or irritability
- loss of interest in life and desire to do anything
- loss of appetite
- sleep-related problems
- rapid weight loss or gain
- showing little interest in the baby.

PND can set in any time within six months of childbirth. If you, or your partner, experience these symptoms please contact your family doctor.

Why do babies cry all the time?

Sometimes babies just want to express themselves. Be honest: don't you feel better after a good cry? Besides, what else can they do to get your attention? It's not as if they can click their fingers, raise their hand, whistle, shout or politely ask you to change their nappy.

If your baby is crying it's a process of elimination to determine what they need. There is even an iPhone application (no, not one of our make-believe ones—a real one) which supposedly tells you what your crying baby needs. We think the $9.99 would be better spent elsewhere, but you may disagree!

The process of elimination

- Is the baby hungry? How long since the last feed?
- Does the nappy need to be changed? Inspect.
- Is the baby too hot or too cold? (Learn how to take your baby's temperature; a thermometer that measures room temp is also a great idea.)
- Does something hurt (tight nappy, clothing tags, body position?)
- Does baby need to be swaddled? Babies love to be wrapped up tight, and learning how to swaddle is an absolute must for every new dad. Master that skill and you're halfway home.
- Does your baby want to be cuddled?
- Does your baby want to be rocked/taken for a walk?
- Is your baby overstimulated? Babies take everything in. Sometimes they do well with lots of commotion. Other times they just want peace and quiet.

If none of these seems to work or help, it's OK to ask your mum or mother-in-law for advice.

You'll learn through experience what you can do to calm your baby. If you're worried because your baby seems listless and does not respond to things that normally calm them, make an appointment to see your doctor right away. Go with your gut feeling.

Remember one of the most all important rules: never shake your baby. If your baby's crying is stressing you out and no one is there to take over, put the baby down in a safe place and walk to another room until you calm down. Your calm body helps your baby calm down.

A crying baby will be frustrating and stressful to a new parent, particularly in combination with sleep deprivation. It's important to realise that crying is the primary way babies communicate; it's also their main source of exercise. If you listen closely, you'll be surprised what they tell you.

Don't worry about spoiling your baby by picking it up all the time—your baby is smart, but not smart enough yet, to manipulate you.

As you can see, it's action stations and all hands on deck in these crazy first few weeks. We've only scratched the surface in terms of what's to come, but those first few weeks set a pattern for how you will work together as parents. Talk, talk and talk some more. Discuss your feelings, about what's working and what's not. If you're both relaxed and happy (as much as you can be at this time), chances are your baby will be too.

Chapter 11

Baby development

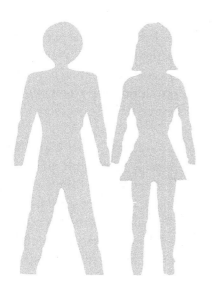

FOR H⚇R

The first few months of having the baby home can seem like all work and no play. Many guys find the first few weeks and months difficult in terms of bonding with the baby. It just doesn't feel as if there is much happening, and the level of interaction is relatively low. Obviously there is plenty that dad can be doing to help out and be involved, but much of that doesn't help him bond with the baby.

Why is it that many blokes need something in return from the baby? Earlier on we wrote about how nutrition and exercise helps a baby develop, and that knowledge may help some guys feel that they are making a valuable contribution to the baby's development. But what about once the baby has come out?

The best thing dads can do with their babies is play with them, interact with them and show affection to them. These are vital ingredients of the mental and emotional development of every baby. How many guys know how to do this instinctively? Not many.

It's important for you to let him have time alone with the baby and establish his own play routines. If you find it difficult to not be a helicopter mum hovering around telling him what to do, take a deep breath and get out of the house for an hour or two. Let them be alone together. It will build his confidence and give you some valuable time off. Remember, blokes like to push their baby's boundaries and are often OK with letting them fall over, take small risks and generally learn things the hard way. Believe it or not, that's actually a good thing for your baby—as long as he's not letting your baby crawl around on the freeway, hang out with large black dogs solo, light his own cigarettes or practise walking on bench tops, bite your tongue and let him be.

Simply ensuring that your baby is well fed and has a clean nappy does little to build the language learning skills or provide the emotional support the baby needs. So if that's the extent of Dad's role, it does little to help the bonding process.

Ask most guys what their one-month-old baby is doing and he'll say, 'Sleeping, crying, eating or pooing.' What's junior really up to, and how is he or she developing on a weekly basis? How can dad help, and follow his baby's development?

In this chapter we will show him what activities he can do with the baby, how he can look for signs of development and understand when the baby is actually interacting with him even though this may not mean being able to catch a footy or bowl a cricket ball.

FOR H♂M

When your nipper enters the world you'll ask yourself one big question: 'What do we do now?' Pre-season trials are over and now the season proper begins.

Now that you're a dad you'll have lots of people ask you if you've bonded with the baby. Some people talk about having an instant connection with their baby the first moment they meet—love at first sight, perhaps. That's great, but the reality for a lot of people is that bonding can take time. It may take weeks, months, maybe even as long as a year, and while you're waiting for it to happen you may feel guilty and question your ability to be a good dad. But don't worry, as the baby grows you'll come to love that little one like crazy.

During the first year your baby is developing in many ways—physically, cognitively and emotionally—but in the early months the most important aspect of development is their sense of confidence in and connection with their parents. It's not just about the baby, though; getting involved and interactive with your baby sets a tone for your future relationship.

Expressing emotion isn't easy for everyone. Getting used to telling your baby you love them from very early on makes it feel natural when they're a bit older. Telling your child that you love them and having them return the compliment is one of the greatest feelings any parent can have.

It's important for you to have time alone with your baby and establish your own play routines. If your partner finds it difficult to not hover around telling you what to do, nudge her out of the house for an hour or two so you and your baby can be alone together. It will build your confidence and give her some valuable time off.

In fact, we think this is a key step. It's bloody hard to do anything with someone looking over your shoulder ready to intervene at the first whiff of an 'error'. It does two things: it prevents you from pushing the boundaries and it prevents you learning from your mistakes. Everyone, including your partner, has put on a nappy backwards. Everyone has put a head through an arm hole and an arm through a leg hole. As long as you're careful, sensible and caring—and follow the major rules, like never shake the baby—you need to have time to make the mini mistakes on your own.

Ship your partner off for a lap of the block or a coffee with the girls or a movie. When she goes do everything that you can to have an enjoyable time, but keep it as simple as possible. Have everything looking respectable when she comes back, so she is happy to let you have another crack at it next week.

Baby development

The following is merely a guide to baby development. Not all babies develop at the same time and rate, so the time frames might be slightly different for your baby. If you're concerned about any aspect of your child's development consult your doctor or paediatrician.

Although your baby will be cooing, babbling and possibly even saying a few choice words (like mama and dada) during the first year, language skills don't really take off until the second year. However, you'll be laying the foundation for these skills, and others, from the day your baby is born.

Tracking your baby's development and playing with them will help the two of you bond. Every week your baby will be doing something new and learning, even though it might seem like all they do is eat, sleep and dirty nappies. Watching your nipper develop is seriously fun and interesting and you can play a significant role in helping them grow physically and mentally.

Week 1

Despite being out and about your baby will spend most of the first two weeks (about 90 per cent of it) asleep, which is brilliant news for you and an opportunity to stockpile as much sleep as possible.

Being outside the womb must be pretty scary for the little one, and your voice and touch are very comforting. Skin-on-skin contact and lots of talking to your baby will make them understand that they're not alone and that you're there to keep them happy, fed, dry, warm and loved. It is believed that babies can recognise their parents' voices from time in the womb, so they can most likely pick you out in a crowd.

They can't understand a word you're saying, so there's no need to talk in a baby's voice. Experts believe babies develop faster if their parents speak normally to them. Get into the habit of telling your baby what you're doing and asking them questions—you may feel that you should be committed to an asylum, but it's good for the baby.

It's not easy to know what to talk about, so here are a few suggestions: sports results, the demise of Australian cricket, the big bang theory, the benefits of running profits and cutting losses, your favourite ten films of all time (and why) and the most influential pop stars of the 1980s. Or you can just start reading books to your baby (it doesn't really matter what books) and telling them you love them. It sounds silly, but if you get used to telling your child you love them now it will become natural and comfortable for you. All kids really need is to know that they are loved—it's a word they really seem to understand from a very young age. You might feel like a goat the first few times you do it, but it's great practice and it will become a habit.

Beware of the tar truck delivery. The first poo will be black and sticky and will look as if someone poured a middy of stout into your baby's trousers. It is called meconium and it's completely normal and completely horrible. Soon the number twos will start looking like mustard with poppy seeds. Get in early with the nappy changes and start acclimatising to poo time. You may also notice some red tinges in the wee. This too is normal and should pass.

At birth infants cannot control their body movements. Most of their movements are reflexes as their nervous system is not fully developed. Think of it as like being really drunk—helpless and in need of physical and emotional support!

Week 2

Your baby's eyes are learning how to zero in on objects. At the moment he or she is near-sighted and has a range of 20–30 centimetres. You might notice when you're feeding that the baby is looking intently at you. That's because you're close enough for them to see your big nose, your goatee and your Michael Clarke signature diamond earring.

You can help build your baby's eye muscles and focal skills by moving your head or a toy from side to side and watching their eyes track it. Reward the baby by letting them watch the footy with you and celebrate with a frosty cold beverage for you and a bottle of mum's finest lactated lager for them. They may even prefer a booby-chino. You will need to improve your dad jokes too. This high level of pun and innuendo has been refined over many months of being a dad, so don't worry. Your time will come.

The umbilical cord will be drying up in preparation for falling off. It looks and smells very ordinary—keep it clean and dry and it will be gone soon.

Your nipper will begin to develop trust in you as you meet their needs (for example, feeding them when they're hungry, changing the nappy when needed or holding them when they cry). Babies cry to express hunger, anger and pain. It is their only way of communicating and it's a sound that will cut through the deepest sleep and get you off the couch even when you just want to lie there forever.

Week 3

The first few weeks of parenting are a complete haze and things like showering seem no longer necessary. You may be lucky and have a sleeper or you may be having a really hard time and getting very little sleep. Either way your baby now recognises your scent, so make sure you're showering regularly and smelling nice! You may feel the baby is willing and able to almost cuddle with you, so whenever you get the chance pick them up and hug away. Putting the baby in bed with you on the weekends is a great way to spend some time.

Week 4

Listen closely to the sounds your baby is making. There is still the wailing cry, but you may also start hearing different sounds: sounds they make when they see you, when they're hungry or when they're feeling uncomfortable. Some people believe that specific noises actually have a meaning, and that by recognising these sounds you will know what your baby wants. We have no idea if it's true or not—but we're as tone deaf as a cricket bat so we were no good at deciphering one sound from another. Unfortunately, your baby is also learning that when he calls out someone comes a-running. They have you worked out already!

Week 5

The baby is starting to get a little more co-ordinated but isn't strong enough to do a great deal. There are lots of baby massage and exercise videos you can buy or rent, and these can be a fun way to interact with your baby and help them start getting used to using their muscles.

Week 6

Around this time your baby may start to smile. They also start to mimic sounds and some movements, so smile at them a lot . . . and they might just smile back. They're not Marcel Marceau just yet but the ability to smile will impress the pants off you.

Activities for weeks 1–6

- Hold your baby often; get the baby used to your touch and smell. Your physical attention builds a sense of safety and security which they need to feel happy.

- They'll be intrigued by your face, so pull faces and talk to them. Introduce new textures to their fingers and skin.

- Hold your baby up to a mirror; this way they can get to know themselves. Point out their features and your features. They can't understand you, but you're laying the foundation for language skills that will develop soon enough.

- Sing songs. Incorporate gentle arm and leg movements. This provides a great opportunity to delve into your old cassette and CD collection. A newborn is the only individual incapable of turning it off so they make a great musical wingman.

- You can help build your baby's neck muscles by lying down on your back, putting the baby face down on your chest with his toes pointing towards your toes and lifting your head up slightly. The baby will try to look at your face, which will make them lift their head, strengthening those neck muscles.

- Change the baby's view; if you're at home, move the baby around so that they can see different things around the house. They will be fascinated by new surroundings but remember, babies can get bored too.

- Get out of the house. It's a great track by Boom Crash Opera and a good suggestion for you and your baby. Whack the baby in a baby carrier or the stroller and just get outside. Whether it's the middle of winter or summer, being outdoors will keep the baby amused and you refreshed and fit. It's very easy to hunker down, but you will start getting cabin fever and so will junior.

Week 7

Sounds, colours and other stimuli will start getting their attention. Objects that make noise, bright colours and movement will start to be interesting. Play with different toys to find the ones that really get their attention. Try to avoid collecting plastic crappy toys; they will become the bane of your existence and they consume empty space like a flesh-eating disorder.

Give your baby plenty of tummy time to start strengthening their neck muscles.

Week 8

Put your baby on his stomach in front of a mirror. Just like you they like to check themselves out, and to do so they need to lift their head up. What more incentive do you need?

By this time your baby will be able to focus on smaller objects and may even be able to grab on to them. Always keep an eye on the baby and make sure any objects within reach aren't so small that they could choke on them.

Week 9

This week is music appreciation week. Your baby is enjoying new sounds and you may notice him or her watching your mouth move as you speak. They take in everything that you do. Put the baby in a sling or baby carrier and rock out to a few of your favourite tunes when it's just the two of you. Is your baby a Michael Jackson or a Cold Play kid?

Start reading the baby a nursery rhyme book every day. It's hard to believe, but reading to a baby helps them develop a vocabulary of words that they can recognise and come to understand.

Week 10

Enjoy the fact that your baby is still not mobile by taking him or her out with you to dinner or wherever other people are. Kids seem to like noise and lots of action, but that's not to say they would enjoy a rock concert. Watch how your baby can pick you out in a crowd of faces—he or she knows exactly who you are.

Week 11

Your baby will start to 'wake up' now and sleep less during the day.

Week 12

Three months old already! Now your baby is honing his or her motor skills; they can control their hands and arms a little better and can hold their own hands and suck on their fingers. Make sure to trim their nails so they can't scratch themselves—fingers have a habit of ending up in eyes!

Activities for weeks 7–12

- Encourage tummy time. This will help to develop your baby's neck and upper body muscles. It's important to supervise tummy time and always make sure your baby is on his or her back when you put them to sleep (to avoid the possibility of sudden infant death syndrome, or SIDS).

- Stimulate rolling over. Babies usually learn to roll over at somewhere between four and six months of age, but you can start encouraging yours to roll over before then. Rolling helps build muscles and keeps your baby entertained. Also, it is a great party trick for your mates.

- Sound identification: record the sounds of normal activities—a dog barking, a door opening, footsteps—and play them back for your baby while explaining what they are. Record your baby's laughter and play it back to him or her. Most mobile phones have a voice recorder and loudspeaker.

- Read a book; simple picture books with lots of colours are best. Your baby may not be very interested but introducing reading can't be a bad thing. It's tempting to put on a baby DVD, but your baby will get more out of you interacting with them. New research shows that those baby DVDs might do more harm than good. Buy a fish bowl instead!

- Bubble time. Get a bubble maker and blow bubbles at your baby. Let the baby practise catching and hitting them—it's good for hand-eye coordination and motor skills.

- Peek-a-boo. Your baby won't begin to develop 'object permanence'—the idea that something doesn't cease to exist when it is out of sight—just yet, but you can start to introduce the concept now. Try peek-a-boo: put a blanket over your face and then remove it so your baby can see that you're still there. This is your chance to be the comedian you always believed you were.

- Let baby play alone. Although you're a crucial part of your baby's development, helping may sometimes mean just letting the baby play alone for a while. Children learn a great deal from playing on their own and exploring the world in the way that they feel driven to. Despite what you may think, your baby is constantly assessing the world and determining their own laws of the universe.

Chapter 12

Babies and pets

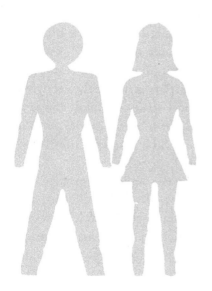

FOR H♀R/H♂M

The following chapter is really only relevant for those of you with pets or considering getting a pet. If that's not you, skip to The end.

When you think about it, there isn't much difference between pets, blokes and babies. We all need looking after, are often incapable of feeding ourselves and require a great deal of love and attention. We also all whine a lot, are poorly toilet trained and tend to create a mess.

When we sat down to write this book we didn't even think about writing a chapter on pets and babies. As renters in Sydney's eastern suburbs it's pretty difficult to have a dog or cat, so a pet was one thing we didn't have to have to worry about.

As fate would have it we were introduced to vet extraordinaire Dr Katrina Warren, whom you've no doubt seen on TV. Katrina, as you can imagine, is passionate about all things pets and has a menagerie of dogs, cats and birds plus a new baby. Katrina told us that pets and babies are a real issue for many couples. Apparently there is a phenomenon known as 'fur babies', which refers to couples with pets but no kids. So if you have a fur baby, how will it be affected by a real baby?

After a discussion with Katrina on the subject of pets, blokes and real babies, we felt it was a topic well worth exploring. All the information below was gleaned from Katrina and her website www.drkatrina.com.au. We've asked Katrina to give us the inside running on pets and babies—how to prepare them, what to do when the baby comes home and how to co-exist safely. So here it is.

Why you should prepare your pets for the baby

The media loves to report on attacks on children involving the family pet. The stories are often horrific and have disastrous consequences for the children, the parents and the animal concerned. Personally, we always think of the bigger, more aggressive beasts when it comes to this subject, but it would seem even the little mutts, pussies and tweeties can be problematic.

Kids under five years are at the greatest risk of being attacked by their family pet or by a pet known to them, and most attacks happen at the family home. You've no doubt started taking measures to childproof your home. If you have a pet you should include it on the list of childproofing things to do.

Start early

As we've already mentioned, pets are like blokes. They are territorial and need quite a bit of time to adjust to major changes around the house. Imagine if you didn't tell your man that he was going to be a dad and one day bought a baby home, throwing his life into a kind of chaos he didn't expect and wasn't prepared for. Chances are he would be resentful towards you and the baby. The same goes for your pets. They too need to go through an assimilation program, so it's best to start working on both pet and partner early on in your pregnancy.

Start reducing your pet's dependence on you

If you spend more time with Fido than your partner does you may need to start reversing the roles. Just as your partner will start needing to adjust to being number two so that you can focus on the baby, the family pet also needs to start adjusting to less 'you time'. Just like your man, your pet may actually get jealous, feel resentful of the baby or get depressed because he feels starved of your attention. We're not sure what's worse, a whiney man or a whiney pet, but you get the picture.

It's a shame pets can't talk. If they could, you could sit them down with you partner and give them a good talking to at the same time:

> 'OK guys, when the baby gets home I'm going to be flat out feeding and looking after me and the baby. You're going to have to get used to the fact that I can't spend as much time as I'd like to with both of you. Sam, if you could pick up your undies, do the laundry and keep the bathrooms clean that would really help. Scooby, if you could try not to poo in the backyard that would be a real bonus. I don't want to hear any whining at the back or bedroom door when you're hungry or need attention. You're both big boys now so toughen up. If not, you'll both be sleeping in the dog house. Got it? Good. Sam, take Scooby for a walk and pick up the poo in the backyard, there's a good dog.'

Subtle adjustments to his domain

Just like the way we suggested making subtle changes to his domain rather than putting all his toys in the garage or tearing down the spare room in the first week of pregnancy, you'll need to do the same with your pets. Where will they sleep? Will there be areas (like the nursery) that will be out of bounds? Will you be putting in gates or sealing the doggy door shut? The last thing you want is a pet (or partner) whining when you get the baby home. Decide what changes need to be made to their space and start adjusting them to it slowly.

Bad habits die hard

What's your dog like to walk? Is he a high energy or unpredictable hound? If he's uncontrollable now, how's he going to be when you're also trying to manage your baby? You might have to break him and your man in with some trial walking with an empty pram. Other bad habits, such as jumping up on you or visitors, may also need to be nipped in the bud.

Other reasons men and pets are similar

You should start familiarising them all with the sound of a crying baby. Katrina recommends playing recordings of crying babies to pets and we recommend you do the same for your man. Start running fire drills in the middle of the night with your clock radio blaring crying baby sounds. Get him used to getting out of bed and heading towards the nursery and to broken sleep. Dogs have sensitive hearing, men have selective hearing—each needs to be acclimatised and addressed!

Get them both familiarised with the products and smells of the nursery. Let them in at the same time to have a good old sniff around. While you're explaining the ins and outs of nappies, lotions, wipes and the like to him, let Fido have a sniff around the cot, change table and any other new items.

Have a plan in case the baby comes early. Your man needs instructions on what to do in an emergency or premature birth and you'll need a plan for your pets. Who will look after them while you're in the hospital (friends or a kennel?). Let's hope your man can fend for himself!

Make sure they are all healthy. Get claws trimmed and all males neutered, and ensure that they are clean and disease free!

> **FACT**
>
> There are as many tigers in the US as there are in the wild in the world, and less than 10 per cent of them are in professional zoos or sanctuaries. The remainder are kept as

domestic pets. The above advice is not meant for big cats including tigers, lions, cheetahs, lynxes or bobcats. If you do have one lurking around the backyard, feed your partner to it and then call your local zoo officials.

It's not just the baby who can get hurt!

It's not just the babies who can be terrorised by pets. What about the pets? Kids love to play with animals and how are they to know that an HB pencil wasn't designed to take a dog's temperature? More than one pet has been washed by being flushed down a toilet, put in a dish washer or washing machine and dried off in a microwave. These are innocent acts that wouldn't be so cute if it was the dog that flushed the child down the toilet!

Ears, tails and eyes are on the endangered list, and it's little wonder Fido and Garfield occasionally lash out in self-defence. Regardless of how long you've had your pets and how much trust you have in them, Katrina recommends that you NEVER leave any child under the age of eight alone with a pet. Her mantra is separate or supervise: if you can't be in the same room at the same time, your pet needs to moved outside or into a different room from your child.

Katrina also recommends that you shouldn't introduce new pets (cats, dogs, tigers and bears) to the family when children are under the age of five.

You filthy animal

Blokes, babies and pets can all be quite disgusting, and can and do display pretty ordinary levels of personal hygiene. What parts of this do you need to worry about?

- Worms (from your pets and from others): ensuring that your pets are wormed regularly isn't too difficult, but you have no way of knowing if others are.

- Scratching: keep nails/claws trimmed and clean.

- Toxoplasmosis: Katrina told us that many pregnant couples have given away their cat due to a fear of toxoplasmosis. It sounds more like something Superman uses to regenerate his super powers but it can be a health risk to an unborn baby. Basically, it is an infection with a parasite called 'Toxoplasma gondii' which infects warm-blooded animals including humans. Usually it causes no symptoms, and many people will already have come into contact with this parasite without knowing it, and will have built up immunity. However, it can cause serious disease in unborn babies. Fortunately this is rare, but pregnant women should follow simple precautions to minimise the risks of infection. It can be caught by eating contaminated raw or partly cooked meat or by using contaminated food utensils that have been in contact with raw meat or infected cat faeces. Avoid handling or eating uncooked or undercooked meat, always wear gloves when cleaning the litter tray and make sure the trays are cleaned and disinfected daily. Katrina insists that there is no need to your throw pussy out with your breaking waters but it's very important you follow these hygiene tips when it comes to dealing with litter trays and feline fecal matter.

- Basic hygiene: we can't believe we even need to write this, but Katrina's main advice when it comes to hygiene and pets is to always wash your hands after playing with any animal, to not let them lick your kids on the face (and vice versa) and to never pick up dog or cat poo with your bare hands. And if your backyard is full of 'animal landmines' (poos), dispose of them before Junior is able to pick them up and eat them.

Pets do not make good Christmas presents

Pets do not make great gifts. There is an alarming rate of pet abandonment as a result of people not being prepared to cope with pets and kids. According to the RSPCA, far too many pets given as Christmas presents are abandoned or put into the pound by Easter. Don't underestimate how much work a pet can be and how quickly your kids can tire of having to look after them. Having a pet is like having a child: a lot of work and a long-term commitment.

If you'd like more information on pet and baby safety visit Katrina's website, which is brimming with loads of great advice and activities for parents and kids.

Conclusion

Assuming you started reading this book when you started trying to get pregnant, and managed to do so quickly, we've covered a year in your life. Not any ordinary year, but a truly extraordinary one in which you grew a baby, gave birth and managed to make it through the first three months of being a parent. Surely there cannot be a more action-packed, life-changing 12 months in anyone's life. If, however, you aren't pregnant yet and have read the book we hope you haven't been scared off!

It's really not feasible that any book can do justice to those 12 months or cover all the possibilities that could arise. To do so would require a tome of epic proportions and the paper usage alone would cause public outrage in this eco-friendly world.

Talk to your friends and family who have been through pregnancy, birth and parenting. Listen to their stories, tips and advice, but remember that you'll develop your own parenting style. It's OK to be scared, to mess things up, to make mistakes, to cry like a baby and just wish you'd stayed single, foot loose and fancy free. No one tells you that this parenting caper is bloody hard work and an assault on your relationship—apart from us that is!

As we've tried to reinforce throughout the book, we, the authors, aren't any more expert than you or anyone else who has been aboard the parenting rollercoaster. Believe us when we say we've stuffed up with the best of them, made more mistakes than most and have cried like babies on many occasions.

We wish you well in your journey and hope that you can remember to see the lighter side of things when you are covered in vomit or poo, are walking the streets at 4 am with a screaming baby, haven't slept in days, despise your partner, have sore nipples, get a flat tyre on the stroller, have to watch The Wiggles for the four-hundredth time in a week, feel fatter than a house or just like the world is about to end. We've all been there—hell, we're all still there. It never ends but it's all worth it. After all, would you rather be 22 again, travelling the world with not a care in the world other than where you'll be going out drinking tonight? Don't answer that.

It's time to close this book for the last time, track down your partner, tell them how much you love them and make out like crazy . . . and then do it again—you'll feel all the better for it.

Sam and Troy

Index

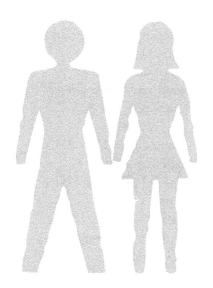